Peace Between the Sheets

Peace Between the Sheets

Healing with Sexual Relationships

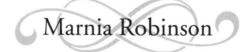

Marnia Robinson

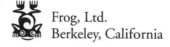

Frog, Ltd.
Berkeley, California

Published by Frog, Ltd.

Frog, Ltd. books are distributed by
North Atlantic Books
P.O. Box 12327
Berkeley, California 94712

Cover design, photography, and book design by Maxine Ressler
Author photo by Kim Leibowitz

Printed in the Canada

Although anyone may find the suggestions in this book useful and beneficial, they are not intended as a diagnosis, prescription, recommended treatment, or cure for any specific problem, whether medical, emotional, psychological, social or spiritual. This book was written for educational purposes only and not designed to replace therapy or consultation with a qualified professional. All names have been changed, though stories have been taken from real-life discussions and experiences.

North Atlantic Books' publications are available through most bookstores. For further information, call 800-337-2665 or visit our website at www.northatlanticbooks.com.

Substantial discounts on bulk quantities are available to corporations, professional associations, and other organizations. For details and discount information, contact our special sales department.

Library of Congress Cataloging-in-Publication Data
Robinson, Marnia, 1954-
  Peace between the sheets : healing with sexual relationships / by Marnia Robinson.
      p. cm.
Includes index.
  ISBN 1-58394-087-1 (pbk.)
  1. Sex. 2. Orgasm. 3. Man-woman relationships. 4. Intimacy (Psychology) I. Title.
  HQ21.R7515 2003
  306.7--dc22   2003017717

1 2 3 4 5 6 7 8 9 TRANS 08 07 06 05 04 03

This book is lovingly dedicated to Gary Bruce Wilson,
whose courage, knowledge, and open heart
finally brought it to life

Table of Contents

PART II: How   147

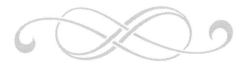

Introduction

THE BOOK YOU ARE HOLDING IS NOT A TYPICAL RELATIONSHIP manual. Instead of rehashing conventional wisdom about love and sex it presents a unique combination of ancient wisdom and modern science. It explains how we are imprisoned by the unconscious script of the primitive part of our brain and outlines a radical prescription for freeing ourselves: making love differently. The goals are to heal the disharmony between the sexes and tap the most profound gifts of union—consistently. As I gathered the material within, it confirmed my deepest suspicions even while it aroused my intense resistance. Ultimately it changed the way I saw sexual relationships, passion, romance, addiction, and antagonism between lovers.

If you are a mammal and not in a coma, your so-called primitive brain has had far more say about your intimate relationships than has your free will. You may have acted upon its primal urgings and wondered at the resulting heartache—ranging from explosions of anger and infidelity to dreary stagnation. Or you may have retreated into celibacy to avoid these pitfalls—in many cases accompanied by your chosen addiction. Unfortunately, neither path offers the deep satisfaction of the middle path that lies between impulse and abstention.

This path has been around for thousands of years—though our physical design ensures that we generally overlook it.

In explaining why we would wish to master this middle path of conscious sexual union I will try to recapture my initial resistance to the idea and share some of the evidence that changed my mind.

"If It Ain't Broke, Don't Fix It"

It is broke. Intimate relationships are not faring well. "Marriage trends in the United States in recent decades indicate that Americans have become less likely to marry, and that fewer of those who do marry have marriages they consider to be 'very happy.'"[1]

I was a bridesmaid in three weddings, as well as a bride in my own, and twenty years later, all of those marriages have ended in divorce. My experience mirrored others' rocky love lives. Between 1960 and 2000, the percentage of divorced adults quadrupled.[2] Emotional separation between couples (married or unmarried) is widespread, and staying married is no guarantee that the fundamental problem has been solved. Marriages are often miserable ghosts of their once affectionate, romantic, mutually supportive states.

I think I personally tried all the mainstream recommendations for healing disharmony in intimate relationships: better communication, finding the right mate, more passion, loving my inner child, negotiation, and so forth. These remedies do not arrest relationship deterioration once trouble starts because they are addressing symptoms of a more fundamental problem. The real problem is right under our noses. It has always been there, but now that church and state have lost the power to keep us married, it is even more glaring. Once we acknowledge it the solution is evident.

The trouble begins with sex. Not exciting sex versus boring sex, as most of us have been led to believe, but rather sex itself. After all, platonic friendships between men and women work just fine. The trouble starts when we become lovers. And what else begins then? For everyone? The pursuit of orgasm.

Passion seems like our best friend—often the one indisputably *good* thing about an otherwise dysfunctional relationship. However, hot sex has hidden costs that doom us to disharmony as time passes. Orgasm can become our relationship's worst enemy, and we are intended by evolution to disregard the link between the intoxicating cause and the dismal effects.

Our blind spot is coming into focus, however. New advances in brain science (neuroendocrinology) are revealing that emotional alienation between lovers may have less to do with communication or compatibility than we thought and more to do with a section of our brains called the pleasure/reward center. Evolutionary biology, the force that encourages us to replicate ourselves as often as possible, currently exploits this brain mechanism by ensuring that we receive a powerful neurochemical "reward" when we engage in hot sex ... or even think about it. That pay-off feels as though it is promoting bonding at the moment of orgasm, but the blast triggers further neurochemical changes that, over time, push us apart from our lovers.

Basically, evolutionary biology has subverted human will to its single-minded purposes of duplicating more genes and promoting genetic variety. Once you understand the means biology uses, its unsuspected effects upon you, and a practical option, you will be in a better position to choose whether you wish to remain under its command—or take control.

"But Sex with Orgasm Is Normal"

True. But so is the middle path that the ancients advocate. The approach of making love frequently and contentedly, without orgasm (as we currently know it), has been around for thousands of years. The reason it first strikes us as bizarre is because we have never experienced its many benefits. Also, we are so deeply hypnotized that we fail to see how much damage biology's strategy currently inflicts on our relationships.

Perhaps you have heard of the Coolidge Effect. Scientists have shown (and you have to suspect that it gets lonely in the lab with experiments like this one . . .) that if you sexually exhaust a male rat with one female, his body chemistry will shut him down. If he were a guy, he would head for the La-Z-Boy toting the remote. As a result of his changed body chemistry (fatigue), Miss Rat will look totally uninteresting to him.[3] However, if he is placed near Miss Ratty (a new female), his exhaustion will mysteriously fade long enough for him to gallantly fulfill his fertilization duties. This is known as the Coolidge Effect.

Does the Coolidge Effect show up in human behavior, too? I recall a conversation I once had with a man who had grown up in sensual Los Angeles. "I quit counting at 350 lovers," he confessed, "and I guess there must be something terribly wrong with me because I always lost interest in them sexually so quickly. Some of those women are really beautiful, too." At the time of our chat his third wife had just left him for a Frenchman and he was discouraged. She had mysteriously lost interest in him.

Gandhi himself apparently exploited the power of the Coolidge Effect. It is rumored that while he was fasting to protest British colonialism he invigorated himself by sleeping between a pair of virgins (new fertilization opportunities). He had long since given up sex with his wife, of course, in favor of celibate spiritual practice. History has not recorded whether Mrs. Gandhi conducted a similar experiment to raise her spirits in the absence of her husband's attentions.

Biology certainly plays its genetically-driven tricks on females, too. Women are more prone to be unfaithful during the fertile days of their menstrual cycles.[4] They are also more likely to have orgasm (which improves the chances of conception by retaining more sperm in their reproductive tract[5]) not with loving, sensitive men, but with men whose features are symmetrical (indicating sound genetic structure) even though they make worse-than-average mates.[6]

Until now, most of us have either engaged unthinkingly in impulsive sexual behavior, or put a damper on our own sex drive and reduced our analysis of humankind's plight to moral judgments of others. We would be wiser to understand, with compassion, how we are being manipulated and change course. After all, supplies of Frenchmen and virgins are limited.

Think about it. Evolutionary biology has little use for relationship harmony. As Richard Dawkins explained in *The Selfish Gene*,[7] all life can be viewed as nothing more than competing forms of DNA replication machinery. From this perspective, cockroaches are more successful than humans. And, it is apparent from our inherited behaviors that biology found more benefit in numerous genetic opportunities than in partners cuddling up in blissful sanity.

But here is the headline news: *we are not obliged to follow this evolutionary imperative.* Indeed, as a species we would be wise to choose our procreation opportunities with greater foresight. And as individuals, we are better off in harmonious relationships with high levels of trust than in mindless mating dances. Most of us sense this. Years ago, I happened upon the results of a reader survey in *Playboy* magazine that had asked, "What makes for the best sex?" The answer that received the greatest percentage of votes was "being deeply in love with your partner."

Decades later, I can finally explain why those readers were correct. The gains from caring deeply about another person are profound. Not only do such feelings change our outlook on life for the better, they also have positive physiological effects. These gifts include improved physical health, reduced stress, and even rejuvenation.

Sexual intimacy that can do all this is truly great sex. And to experience it continuously all we have to do is stay in love. Indeed, if logic ruled, we would stay in love. The problem arises when biology rules and the aftereffects from its incentive plan (unbridled passion) separate lovers. As one friend so eloquently put it, "Evolution doesn't give a rat's ass about love, fidelity or companionship."

A way to defy biology's dictates has been around for millennia. I think of it as an all-you-can-eat diet of your *other* favorite things about intimacy: physical affection, satisfying lovemaking, mutual trust, emotional closeness, and the opportunity for personal growth/healing. I suspect that the approach I now use when I make love is similar to that recorded by the ancient Chinese Taoists, among others. Yet Western minds generally prefer to isolate the fundamentals of these traditions using an analytical, experiential approach. So while acknowledging with deep gratitude the signposts left by these early teachers, I will present the material as I learned it—through a combination of esoteric clues, trial and error, and analyzing new scientific discoveries.

"You Just Have to Find the Right Person"

 Here are the words of a monogamous husband and father of thirteen children who was a shrewd observer of human nature:

> In life this preference for one [lover] to the exclusion of all others lasts in rare cases several years, oftener several months, or even weeks, days, hours.... Every man feels what you call love toward each pretty woman he sees, and very little toward his wife.... [And] even if it should be admitted that Menelaus had preferred Helen all his life, Helen would have preferred Paris....   —Leo Tolstoy[8]

More than a century ago, Tolstoy recognized that periods of passion in his marriage were inevitably followed by angry eruptions between his wife and him. If they were not openly hostile to each other they numbed themselves to cope with their emotional distress. He smoked and drank too much and his wife drove everyone to distraction with trivial household and child-related agitation. After years of observation he realized that lust toward one's beloved was the culprit. But the ancient texts revealing another way to make love were still virtually unknown in his time. So he only saw two miserable options: sexual abstinence within his marriage or lust followed by intense irritation.

If anything, the problem he portrayed is growing more pronounced. Look what happened to Pamela Anderson and Tommy Lee—or Billy Bob Thornton and Angelina Jolie. For most of us "finding the right person" means finding someone who jolts our brain chemistry into the red zone. But even less passionate couples who base their unions on the traditional marriage deal are splitting up with alarming frequency.

The erosion of monogamy *is* due to chemistry, but not chemistry in the usual sense. Once again neuroscience has turned up a vital clue in a rodent experiment. Prairie voles are mouse-like critters that mate for life—which their montane vole-cousins do not. Because of this striking difference, scientists were able to figure out that monogamy is linked to certain neurochemicals. When scientists block these neurochemicals' effects in the prairie vole, it blithely switches to casual sex. In other words, neurochemistry is closely related to the strength of relationships. For example, at the right levels and locations, the neurochemical oxytocin can make us want to stay together without even trying.

We can only keep the oxytocin flowing if we remain openhearted. The lust cycle, however, carries us from intense desire to uneasy satiation, and back to intense desire, just as Tolstoy observed. These emotions make us greedy, needy, cranky, and defensive, rather than openhearted. Bang!—pardon the pun—the neurochemistry of romance succumbs to the neurochemistry of uneasiness and separation.

Desire is fine in temperate doses. But blind impulse tends to transform us humans from loyal prairie voles into promiscuous montane voles. That might not matter to many people these days, except that scientific research also shows that we humans are healthier and happier in harmonious pairs.

So before you abandon another mate try the approach to sex outlined in this book. The results may amaze you. Though I was initially drawn by the concept's promise of greater relationship depth, the first change I noticed was a distinct improvement in my health. Chronic yeast and urinary tract infections simply stopped—for good—and I have not needed a doctor for anything in over a decade.

My fiancé Will is also pleased with the healing he has experienced. He is more energetic and productive, has released a long-term addiction, and no longer requires a prescription antidepressant. Two years into our relationship he is delighted by its sanity, playfulness, lovingness and increasing closeness.

Our health improvements and harmony are aligned with claims in various ancient sacred-sex texts. But Will, a long-time student of human sciences, is more intrigued by the light that modern science sheds on these phenomena. Will's research, which I include, suggests that the early Chinese Taoists, Tibetan Buddhists, Tantra sages, and even pre-Roman Christians, all of whom advised a less heated, more altruistic approach to sex, were shrewder than most modern sexologists.

Peace Between the Sheets

 This book has two parts. The first is about *why* I changed the way I made love. It will confront various cherished assumptions of most readers, as it recommends avoiding masturbation as much as possible, learning to make love without conventional orgasm, healing all alienation from the opposite sex, and putting relationship harmony before the usual agendas for sexual intimacy.

Above all, it recommends altruism in the bedroom—not an easy feat, as your brain chemistry is all set up to bestow on you a mighty reward for being as selfish as possible during sex. However, that neurochemical reward does not lead to increased well-being, while the alternative does.

Nothing will convince you of the validity of this approach as effectively as giving it a try. Therefore, the second part of the book tells *how* I went about it. It includes various practical tips as well as a series of simple activities for couples wishing to circumvent their unconscious biological programming. The key concept is to nurture each other while you go through a couple of weeks of withdrawal. The resulting improvements in your neurochemistry actually reduce cravings for orgasm (and any other addictions). This natural shift enables you to settle into a pattern of lovemaking that can radically benefit your health and relationship.

This book is a road map. It could not have been compiled or published without the generous help of many friends, lovers, friends of lovers, and lovers of friends. Some, like Mary Sharpe, were brave enough to try the ideas. She in turn inspired me by returning to university at Cambridge to compose a thesis on sexuality and the sacred in connection with an advanced degree in religion. Others helped by critiquing my ideas at every turn, contributing their own gems of experience and inspiration, building websites, looking after me as I moved back and forth between Europe and the United States, drawing pictures, proofreading, editing, tracking down references, solving graphics crises, and simply loving me even though my unusual vocation made no sense to them whatsoever. I am deeply indebted to this chain of enthusiasts, loved ones and guardians, which stretches from California to Bavaria with special links in Arizona, Belgium, England, Florida, Italy, and New York.

I would also like to thank the funny folk whose witticisms about the gender gap I could not resist adding to the text. Many of the jokes serve as grim reminders of the current state of affairs. From my new perspective, however, humanity's circumstances are genuinely laughable. We have unwittingly allowed a mindless neurochemical reward mechanism to push us around for ages. As it turns out, there was a better way all along. Now that the planet is teeming with under-fed, under-loved human beings, it is time to get serious about mastering that better way. While I admit that I do not yet have all the answers, I hope you will find some helpful clues within. At the very least you will be equipped to avoid mankind's unsuspected obstacle to deep union as you work toward creating the intimate relationship for which your soul yearns.

I don't mind women leaving me ... but they always have to tell you *why*.
—Richard Pryor

—Marnia Lynn Robinson, 2003

Part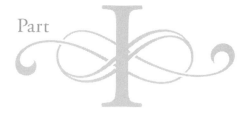

Why

There is a principle which is a bar against all information, which is proof against all arguments and which cannot fail to keep a man in everlasting ignorance. That principle is contempt prior to investigation.

—Herbert Spencer, nineteenth-century British philosopher

Chapter 1

Why Do
We Fall Out
of Love?

HAVE YOU EVER FALLEN IN LOVE WITH SOMEONE WHO LOVED you back? What an experience! Suddenly the world begins to make sense. With higher voltage you flow with inspired ideas. Life takes on a rosy glow, and the wings and halo of your loved one are clearly visible. Yet, if things take their normal course, you will soon look back on this brief interval of heightened awareness as the honeymoon period, and regard it as a sort of . . . deception.

It is not a deception. Something quite real is going on. A complete circuit of energy is flowing between your hearts, and it is actually making you more energetic, expanding your perception, and profoundly improving your body chemistry. When humanity learns to follow this spiraling energy upward all the way we will tap into something truly profound. According to various spiritual traditions across the globe this flowing circuit between lovers is nothing less than a path to enlightenment.

For now, however, most of us never make it anywhere near the penthouse. Instead we get off somewhere around the third floor and swiftly begin that familiar downward spiral into the mundane . . . too often followed by a nosedive into the basement. This happens because the physical part of us is operating on biological autopilot and we have assumed its will is our own.

My education about healing relationships began with just such a crash. In 1986 my sister, weary of watching the turnover in my love life, gave me a book entitled something like *Marrying the Man of Your Choice*. The book insisted that I needed to write a detailed description of my ideal mate. So I did.

Sure enough he showed up within a year. Not only that, a couple of months before Russ and I met, a psychic at a party assured him that he would meet me by a certain date. She told him my age, my profession, the element of my astrological sign, and several other surprisingly accurate things. We met at a conference in New York City two days before the date the psychic named. It certainly *felt* like a heavenly match. However, shortly after conventional sex entered the picture, the relationship blew apart. And every time we tried again, it blew apart again.

It was excruciating to watch a relationship with someone with whom I had experienced such a fated, profound connection crumble despite all efforts to save it. I turned to my inner guidance demanding an explanation, and that same week I ran into my first Taoist lovemaking book. This book explained that there was another kind of ecstasy possible between intimate partners, and the instant I read the descriptions, I knew it was what I had always been seeking in my relationships:

> The valley orgasm [as distinct from the conventional "peak" orgasm] occurs spontaneously in the deep state of relaxation, and it is a very powerful experience which I feel in every cell, every particle of my being as an exquisite, ecstatic melting. The feeling of connection with my partner is profound. My whole being is shared with his, and his with mine, as one flow that knows no boundaries.... I am always in awe of the tremendous power residing in male and female. We are all closer to being gods and goddesses than we think.... There is a sense of all the time in the world, of being in eternity, and of having more and more energy available.[9]

The "rub," of course, was that to find this valley ecstasy one had to pass up conventional orgasm. Russ, however, was very conservative and had no interest in what he considered unconventional sex. Shortly thereafter I was transferred to Europe. Foiled again.

Getting Hooked on Avoiding Orgasm

Years went by and no Eastern sage showed up to instruct me in mystical union. Determined to learn it, I took inspiration from one of my favorite sayings:

> Never be afraid to try something new. Remember, amateurs built the ark. Professionals built the Titanic.

I concluded that I would have to figure out how to motivate another novice to explore this mystery with me. Swiftly I discovered that, even with good intentions, it is not so easy to leave current sexual habits behind. It can be done, though, and the process is surprisingly enjoyable. With sufficient self-motivation, and clear directions (the second half of this book), you will not have to stumble around as I did.

Here is an account of my first attempt to crack the code: I met Alex in a workshop at a spiritual community in Scotland. A deeply spiritual man, he was taking a break from his psychology practice to travel from Canada around the world and visit various inspirational sites. After the seminar we returned to my home on the European continent. Following much discussion we decided to try a non-orgasmic approach to sex.

I had a book, written by a man, with lots of tips on how men could gain mastery over the urge to ejaculate. It recommended tightening the muscles around the prostate gland, clenching the teeth, counting breaths, and various other forceful techniques—all of which I later learned are not nearly as effective as a very gradual, more relaxed approach to sexual intimacy itself.

In any event, Alex insisted that he did not need any instructions. When we made love, however, it was business as usual. That is, he ejaculated. And for the next several days exactly the same thing happened, despite his genuine intention to avoid orgasm. I kept suggesting he study the manual but he was growing increasingly irascible. When I pointed out that, according to the book, his short temper might be due to frequent orgasm itself, he blew.

"You are crazy to suggest ejaculation has a negative effect on men," he bristled. "I'm a psychologist. If that were the case, I would know about it. If you keep talking like this, you're going to be in a mental institution . . . explaining this to your shrink!"

I could see that further argument would just make things worse, and it occurred to me how nice it would be if he just got on the next train! I managed a stony silence.

Finally he exploded, "I can see you are not going to listen to a word I say until I read that book!"

"That's right, Alex," I admitted.

"Okay, what do I have to read?"

I showed him the four or five pages that explained the techniques mentioned above for men to avoid orgasm.

He flipped through the directions and announced, "Let's go try it."

At that point I was ready to give up the whole idea. This rather unchivalrous invitation did not resemble any of my images of a sacred sexuality encounter. Still, I longed to know if the ideas had any merit.

We made love according to the instructions. He clenched and counted and completed the encounter without ejaculating. Then he amazed me by saying, "I do not believe it. I don't feel unsatisfied. I don't have . . . uh . . . blue balls. *Thank you for teaching me this!*" As astonishing as his newfound enthusiasm was, an even greater surprise followed. Over the next twenty-four hours he was a different man. His anger evaporated and his heart opened. Whereas before he had assured me that he did not need a partner because he was on a spiritual path, now he opened up and talked about how much he had always wanted a mate and was confused by his inability to stay in relationship.

The biggest shift of all was that he saw me in a completely different light. No longer did he recommend institutionalization. Instead he said, "You are so spiritual and generous. God must be really proud of you for sticking to this despite so much resistance." I felt transformed also. My heart cracked open with gratitude and I could clearly see his angelic qualities. I remember thinking, "Thank you for showing me this man's true beauty."

I vowed that I had just had my last pointless meltdown with a lover. I could taste the potential for mutual adoration and satisfying intimacy in the new concept and was more determined than ever to master this unconventional approach to sex. At last I was fully motivated.

Tell Me It Isn't True

As it turned out, I had more senseless meltdowns ahead because some of the vital clues for how one eludes biology were missing from the sacred sex manuals I began to devour. Despite thrilling breakthroughs, my results were unstable. Good intentions and lofty aspirations were clearly not enough. Whenever I slipped into old habits the usual relationship disharmony erupted. Hard as it was to accept, orgasm itself seemed to be the culprit. Once I was prepared to consider this implausible hypothesis, I came upon ample evidence of a painful hook embedded in the lure of sexual attraction. It caused partners to pull away from each other.

Remember the movie *When Harry Met Sally*? Billy Crystal said that thirty seconds after making love he wanted to get out of bed and leave. When I asked a partner about it, he replied, "Yeah, I guess that is how most men feel. 'Boom, I'm done! Elvis has left the building. The fat lady has sung. Thank you ... and goodbye.'" Unfortunately, that subconscious urge to get away makes a partner look totally different after sex, even if you do not leave.

A friend once described his first act of intercourse. "I wanted to cry," he told me, "because she was so beautiful and I wanted her so much. But I remember feeling a little disappointed when I saw her body afterward, and her beauty no longer set me on fire as it had done when I first saw it in a haze of passion."

Strange things happen to our perception of each other after the high of orgasm fades. I think of the shift as a hangover—a temporary phase of subtle uneasiness that follows hot sex. Usually we project it onto our partner or the world around us, imagining that he, she, or circumstances over which we have no control have caused our malaise. Here is a quotation from D. H. Lawrence's essay "Pornography and Obscenity":

> Experience teaches that common individuals [have] a disgusting attitude towards sex, a disgusting desire to insult it. If such fellows have intercourse with a woman, they triumphantly feel that they have done her dirt, and now she is lower, cheaper, more contemptible than she was before.[10]

You are probably thinking that such fellows have some serious issues with their mothers. However, I now suspect this hangover problem may be the reason much of humanity bought into weird notions about sex in the first place. If we can feel anxious enough to bolt after sex, we can also feel uncomfortable enough to convince ourselves that the opposite sex is repulsive, that God is punishing us for engaging in sex, or that it is a good idea to cut off girls' genitals as they do in parts of Africa. Even if we do not feel guilty per se, our perception of ourselves and others can shift for the worse. Remember what Hugh Grant said not long after he was caught with Divine Brown in 1995?

> I don't give a f**k about the morality of it.... I didn't care. Everyone's a dirty beast.

Here is another example of a man's urge to leave after orgasmic sex from John Lee's *The Flying Boy:*

> No matter who the woman was, I was as good as gone the moment we made love. It was at that moment that I always touched something taboo—perhaps my mother, perhaps my pain—and I would have to fly away ... I worried and waited for the most appropriate moment to take flight. If I didn't fly away I ran them off. Either way I knew I couldn't be with them.[11]

And consider this dramatic example of deep, sexually-related fear from the father of modern psychiatry, Sigmund Freud:

> Probably no male human being is spared the fright of castration at the sight of a female genital.[12]

Clearly sex is sometimes linked to irrational feelings strong enough to push partners apart. A Taoist master explains:

> Eventually a man can develop feelings of indifference or hate for his sexual partner because he subconsciously realizes that when he [has sex with her] he loses those higher energies that could make him a truly happy man.[13]

Anyone who studies Traditional Chinese Medicine will be familiar with the idea that orgasm has negative consequences. But seldom do we think of it as a psychological, emotional issue. It is time we did.

Subconscious uneasiness can also account for more than relationship drama, because we do not always project our uneasiness onto each other. Consider the words of psychologist Herb Goldberg in *What Men Really Want*:

> The defensive nature of masculinity creates in men a deeply wary and negative experience of the world, which they see as a place where there is never enough power, control, security or independence.[14]

Unlike Freud and Goldberg, I no longer accept that these defensive beliefs are an innate part of the nature of men. However, something universal is causing them. The more I learn, the more I suspect that the sense of lack pervading human experience originates simply in a perceptual shift associated with sex. The implications are huge. As the light went on, I felt like I had just discovered an elephant in my living room that had been there all along, blocking my progress and mindlessly trampling my relationships.

The Hidden Hangover

Finally I accepted that the shift in my partners' perceptions of me, which I had often sensed, was not strictly a product of my issues or even theirs. It was real. But—and here is the most important point in this book—the perceptual shift was also involuntary and preventable. That is, partners could not possibly stop the shift from occurring without addressing the underlying cause.

I read my sacred sex texts again. There it was in black and white: intercourse is beneficial, but orgasm brings with it a host of problems. Symptoms could include feeling drained, irritability, energy imbalance, health problems, and, most significantly, a growing aversion to one's sexual partner.

The world is full of obvious things, which nobody by any chance ever notices.　　　　　　　　—*Sir Arthur Conan Doyle*

The ancient teachings blamed these troubles on semen loss, so most texts claim that only men suffer from negative effects. This explanation proved too simplistic. I was about to learn with certainty that this post-orgasmic distress likewise affects women—altering their perception of their partners dramatically for the worse—though it sometimes takes longer than it does in men. Semen loss is, in fact, virtually irrelevant.

Generally speaking, people are not aware of this hangover. Indeed, biology has us so firmly hooked on the neurochemistry that accompanies orgasmic sex that we only take into account its overpowering, short-term effects. But have you ever fallen in love with total abandon, experienced wonderful lovemaking, been sure you wanted to stay together forever... and then noticed a strange emotional separation developing between you and your lover? Many times we change partners due to this feeling of separation, believing we are victims of incompatibility.

Actually, we are victims of fluctuating neurochemicals. That is, our partner looks irresistible as the brain chemistry of initial sexual attraction pounds between our ears. But the fire of passion sets off subsequent changes in our brain chemistry that, sooner or later, modify our perception of each other for the worse.

The warm glow of love that formerly lit up our world mysteriously sizzles out, leaving disharmony or stagnation in its wake. Like an alcoholic hangover, these changes cloud our outlook on life and even our spiritual perception. This radical perceptual shift may be why one Tantric text refers to orgasm as "the killing of the inner Buddha."[15]

> If a man says something in the middle of the forest and there is no woman around to hear him ... is he still *wrong?*

As explained in the Introduction, sex activates the pleasure/reward mechanism in the limbic system, or primitive brain, to encourage us to procreate. It is the same mechanism acted upon by alcohol, nicotine, and many other recreational drugs. It is easy to turn on, but, alas, this area of the brain is not designed to sustain continual over-stimulation. As I will explain in detail a bit later in the book, excess stimulation causes the pleasure/reward center to put the brakes on. Some of us feel this slow-down as uneasiness, cravings, flatness, or irritability. Others of us just want to get away. Still others feel the desperate need to remodel our partner to meet our amplified needs.

Unfortunately, the emotional effects of the orgasmic hangover linger far longer than those induced by alcohol. In fact, in my experience, lovers' post-orgasm perception can be distorted for as long as two weeks. And it often gets radically worse before the end of that time.

This extended recovery period probably accounts for Orthodox Judaism's recommended two-week abstinence from intercourse each month. It gave partners a chance to restore their inner equilibrium before the next high/low cycle. The rest of us, however, have little chance of connecting this hangover with our sex lives because we rarely pass up sexual activity long enough to observe a full cycle. (And when we go without sex, we are usually troubled by the pain of emotional isolation instead.)

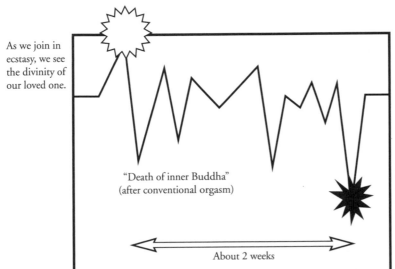

As we join in ecstasy, we see the divinity of our loved one.

"Death of inner Buddha" (after conventional orgasm)

As our hangover kicks in, we see nothing but flaws—or reason for panic.

About 2 weeks

Conventional Orgasm and The Hangover Effect

Many of us have experienced sexually active relationships as brutal see-saw rides until stagnation sets in and/or we break up. I believe this occurs because these unsuspected cycles are at work, overlapping each other. When partners hit low points, each tends to project his or her discomfort onto the other. Typically, he begins to look to her impossibly self-centered, insensitive, and selfish, while she appears to him frighteningly needy, unable to be satisfied, and demanding.

To be sure, these roles are not gender-specific, and the disharmony may take many other forms. When both pull away immediately, we refer to it as a one-night stand. And when both get needy we call it co-dependence.

A Woman's Rule of Thumb: If it has tires or testicles, you're going to have trouble with it.

Usually, however, one lover pulls away while the other desperately seeks to prevent the impending separation by manipulating, over-controlling, or provoking guilty feelings. Wariness breaks the open-hearted trust that was flowing between them. Typically one becomes extremely yin, creating an unhealthy suction in the relationship, while the partner goes extremely yang and pushes the other away.

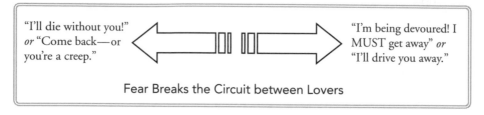

"I'll die without you!" *or* "Come back—or you're a creep."

"I'm being devoured! I MUST get away" *or* "I'll drive you away."

Fear Breaks the Circuit between Lovers

During this hangover period we have a powerful sense that something is not right. And it is not. Unfortunately this syndrome is widespread. So we try to convince each other that our distress is "just life," or it can be fixed by tackling some aspect of ourselves, or avoided by being more selective of our next partner. As the problem keeps recurring, our detailed "must have" lists for future mates grow longer and longer.

It is easy to fool ourselves that conventional sex has nothing to do with our distress because the symptoms rarely show up first as sexual problems. Instead they present themselves as what we perceive to be obvious personality flaws in our lover or ourselves such as addiction, nagging, insensitivity, irresponsible spending, paranoia, stinginess, and compelling attractions to third parties. And so we attack the symptoms instead of the cause.

A Man's Rule of Thumb: No matter how good she looks, some other guy is sick and tired of putting up with her.

Except for the mom and dad in *The Brady Bunch,* I actually know of no couples who have entirely escaped the effects of this fallout for more than the first six months of a committed relationship. Even the happiest-looking marriages soon reveal startling gaps behind the scenes. (See Chapter 6.) It is apparent that there is something more than random bad luck going on. Otherwise at least half of all couples would be blissfully content and making love a lot. They are not.

The Writing on the Wall

As I grasped the dimensions of the problem I realized that others were acknowledging the hangover effect albeit labeling it differently. For example, popular relationship therapist John Gray (*Men are from Mars, Women are from Venus*) teaches that men are like rubber bands, with a pattern of horniness and release followed by periods of emotional alienation from their partners.

I admired his clear articulation of the symptoms when I heard a tape of his. As I recall, his explanation went something like this: "Men, you must get away from women after periods of intimacy, or they will drain you. Women, when that happens, go whine to other women until your man is prepared to sacrifice again for loving contact with you." Though I am grateful for his candor, I think it is unwise to assume that a sense of sacrifice, emotional withdrawal, or draining behavior, are innocuous when they recur in a relationship.

Perhaps you also recall *The Celestine Prophecy* by James Redfield, in which the main character is forbidden to form a relationship with a woman as it would "pull them from the paths of their individual evolution and lead to a hopeless power struggle." And women authors, too, now laud separation. See, for example, *Women, Passion & Celibacy* by Sally Cline, who lists reasons given by various women who opted for celibacy:

> I've had it with men ... no more sexual anxiety ... I wanted a simple life ... sex was boring ... I did it out of spite ... give me companionship not sex ... I needed more time for myself ... my soul was suffering. . . .[16]

Without realizing it, these authors are addressing fallout from the hangover effect that the ancient sexologists warned of. Certainly I have had lovers withdraw "into their caves," as John Gray puts it, after intimacy. And I have found myself in bizarre power struggles with intimate partners that seemed quite senseless a few short weeks later. But is separation, temporary or total, the only way to cope?

Not according to the ancient texts. They insist there is a way to make love without hangovers or alienation. True, convincing someone to forego conventional orgasm is not the easiest sell in the world, but, even early on, I knew it was not impossible either. After all, I had read books written by men advocating it. And, I had seen for myself the benefits to my partners of avoiding orgasm.

As it turned out, convincing my lover not to ejaculate when we made love was not the only obstacle between me and the goal of deeper union. There were still more pieces to this puzzle.

Summary

- The limbic system of the brain, also known as the primitive brain, is programmed to produce a neurochemical buzz that compels us to pursue orgasmic sex, whatever the consequences.
- Orgasm causes subsequent negative physiological changes that can easily last two weeks.
- Orgasm can lead to a shift in perception that often makes our partner look less appealing and may make us want to bolt.
- Ancient teachers of sacred sexuality warn that orgasm has negative consequences such as feeling drained, irritability, energy imbalance, health problems, and, most significantly, a growing aversion to one's sexual partner. They suggest techniques for avoiding ejaculation.

Dave's Story

Before I had a clue what sex was, I knew I wanted to be in love. At age seven, I had a wonderful "love affair." It was divine. It was pure. It was innocent—and completely heart chakra. Amy Willis and I adored each other. When she moved away in third grade I knew I wanted another relationship like that. I was sad she left but still an optimist. I didn't know it was going to be all downhill from there. I've always had a strong attraction to the opposite sex, but I have to admit that after the act of sex entered the picture, love got a lot more complicated.

Thanks to internment in an all-boys prep school, I remained fairly naïve until college. There I faced a most traumatic sexual experience: pregnancy and an abortion. Sex was a wonderful, natural by-product of being in love with someone, but my body clearly wanted to make babies every time I engaged in it. So for that reason and because I was really looking for a lover, not merely a "sexer," I was less apt to engage in casual sex than some of my classmates of the pre-AIDS sexy seventies.

I was a slow learner about some of the facts of life, though. Sex, for me, was the ultimate act of union, so a piece of latex between my lover and me seemed like a major desensitizing compromise. Whenever I had a lover we tried to time our efforts with her cycle or I would withdraw before ejaculating. Although I was not especially promiscuous during the seventies and eighties, I was responsible for more abortions—which caused a lot of heartache for all concerned.

I began to grasp that although there was a lot of pleasure connected with sex—which God must have intended us to have—the planet was painfully over-crowded. And there I was, responsible for a bunch of unwanted pregnancies. I could see it would be a great idea to find states of ecstasy without ejaculating into the woman, but early on I didn't make much progress. As the Beatles put it, the goal was to Come Together.

Finally—after the most tempestuous (read: "passionate") relationship of my life and a set of twins—I was convinced that ejaculating into a partner had definite drawbacks. In the nineties, I began to experiment with avoiding orgasm during intercourse. Ironically, this was made easier because, with the advent of deadly communicable diseases, I was at last wearing condoms.

I still wanted the magical, mystical union of love and I still wanted to please my partner. And my partners still wanted to come during intercourse. I thought I was a very good lover because due to my increasing control they came . . . over and over and over. No longer self-indulgent, I'd become a "pleaser." The big turn-on was her excitement. It's really how I'm received that lights me up. If my lover received me with ecstatic enthusiasm, the pleasure just built and built. And no one got pregnant! Still, if my lover was coming all over me repeatedly all night long, and I wasn't coming at all, an emotional gap ensued. I might add that blow jobs always felt weird to me . . . I don't want to be serviced; I want to be in some sort of mutual bliss. I've always liked to line up my chakras with my lover's—not have my lover somewhere else, like two feet below my chin.

So to pull this rambling to an end, when I read your material suggesting that the way we're using sex links love with fear and results in disharmony, I had to admit that all my relationships had ended in separation. It didn't matter whether I came, or we both came, or only she came. The one possibility I hadn't even thought of, let alone tried, was both of us not coming.

Truth is, I've always wanted a soul mate. But my deepest relationships have not been very healing because there *is* a battle of the sexes going on here. It's kinda cute in a Katherine Hepburn/Spencer Tracy movie, but in my life it has only been painful. In fact, I think the separation of/battle between male and female is the most tragic thing happening on the planet.

I'm a "flaming" heterosexual and, in spite of the love I feel for my brothers, I want to merge with a *woman*. I'm plenty male myself, and it feels like I need the balance of yin energy to complete some . . . circuit. I mean, I feel like a whole man, but that's only half of the equation. Disharmony between the sexes prevents the union I'm longing for. So if sex as conventionally practiced is, indeed, leading to such pathetic results, I figure there must be another way, or . . . it's all just hopelessly screwed up. All I know is there is something tantalizing about the possibility of this last unexplored option being the key to getting off the roller coaster.

Chapter 2

Blind Spots

My girlfriend, Anya, had a new lover. He had grown up in a culture where artificial birth control virtually did not exist, so in order to make love as a teen he had learned to avoid ejaculation. He regarded it as perfectly natural to explore a non-ejaculatory approach to sex with her. She was thrilled. Their lovemaking was sensational, cosmic, lengthy (the phone was once off the hook for four days while I dialed in vain . . .), and her capacity for multiple orgasm as boundless as ever.

But cracks were appearing. A few weeks into her romance she finally called and asked hesitantly, "Do you think there's any chance genital orgasm is a problem for women too. . . ?" I was listening very carefully. During the preceding months I had also finally found a lover who controlled himself easily, but who obviously enjoyed that I climaxed so effortlessly. However, we were certainly not tapping the mystical bliss and union I had read about in the sacred sex books. Instead I was noticing an ugly emotional friction flickering between us.

The issue of the effect of orgasm on women is obscured by the fact that most sexual advice—even esoteric—assumes orgasm is no problem for women because women do not ejaculate semen. For years I fell for this cheerful assumption. Now, however, events were conspiring to bring certain unwelcome truths to my attention.

From this point on Anya and I compared notes like scientists in a laboratory. Regardless of other variables affecting either couple, within a week or two after orgasmic encounters (no matter who climaxed), trouble would erupt. Anya tended to become weepy, oversensitive, ineffective, and discouraged. I tended toward a razor tongue, impatience, pessimism, and analyzing the obviously irreconcilable differences between my lover and myself. Mood swings, which Anya and I had once knowingly blamed on the fallout from our partners' post-ejaculation blues, haunted us both. Why was this happening?

Women's Bumper Stickers:

NEXT MOOD SWING:
6 MINUTES

ALL STRESSED OUT AND
NO ONE TO CHOKE

YOU HAVE THE RIGHT TO
REMAIN SILENT, SO SHUT
UP!

CAUTION: ZERO TO
"BITCH" IN 8 SECONDS

DO NOT START WITH
ME—YOU WILL NOT WIN

Orgasm:
A *Problem* for Women?

Most women are certain that today's focus on genital orgasm is an idea whose time has come. After all, for millennia the heavy boots of patriarchy have stomped about on women's sexuality. Women were relegated to the role of brood mare, forced to let men have their way with them with no attention to their way, and so forth.

As one liberated male explained, "Women have thousands of years of missed orgasms to make up for"—a noble task at which he was diligently beavering away. It is certainly true that many women regard learning to climax as a breakthrough because they previously felt they were missing out on something.

Now, though, Anya and I squirmed as we asked ourselves the same hard questions we had asked about the effects of ejaculation on men. What if some sort of perception shift resulting from orgasm also adversely affected women? How might sexual hangovers manifest in their experience? How about all-around bitchiness? Making him wrong about everything? Reaching for Prozac? Avoiding sex? Feeling unable to cope? Insane jealousy? Fortune hunting? Compulsive shopping, or even kleptomania? Tears and emotional blackmail? Neurotic, needy, controlling mothers—and wounded kids?

Why, it looked like a list of complaints from the minutes of a men's support group meeting. And maybe women could not do much to prevent their bottomless-pit neediness and destructive overreactions unless they, too, addressed the underlying cause of their natural, but avoidable, sense of deprivation. One weary veteran was right on the money:

> Are women crazy, or do I, without knowing exactly how, somehow make them as irrational and volatile as they seem to become after we get involved? They're rarely like that until after we get "serious."[17]

I can stay really loving after orgasm—for about five days max. Then my whole world starts to look ... different, and the only thing I am sure of is that my distress is due to my partner.

What If We've Had it All Wrong?

Tragically, many women have bought into the idea that there is something wrong with them if they do not orgasm easily. Instead of having a problem, they may actually be ahead of the rest of us. Their sexual energy is probably just on strike until they figure out how to use it to deepen their relationships instead of trashing them. Let me quickly add that sexual frustration is not the solution, except insofar as our desire helps pull us toward union. The goal is relearning to use our joint sexual energy in a way that eliminates sexual frustration, without orgasm.

Barry Long, a Tantra teacher in Australia, insists that the vagina does not naturally strive for orgasm. It has to be taught this habit by a society that is obsessed with reaching climax. When it learns to focus on orgasm, it becomes increasingly hard, greedy and predatory. It concentrates on orgasm, not love. This causes deep, inner unhappiness. According to Long, promiscuity is only a desperate search for the love women are not finding through their pursuit of orgasm.[18] Certainly, if

more orgasms were the solution, relationship harmony would be showing a marked improvement in recent years.

> *My last relationship was short. She practically begged me to make*
> *love—and she had an orgasm and everything—but immedi-*
> *ately she wanted to run away ... like she was a guy or some-*
> *thing. A few weeks later, after she slowly warmed back up, we*
> *did it again, and she seemed to have a ... fine time again. Then,*
> *only a few days later, she informed me that "orgasm was a petty*
> *experience" compared with her spiritual practice. In fact, she*
> *told me she was afraid she could get really hooked on sex. I remem-*
> *ber thinking to myself how horrible that would be.*
>
> *And that was pretty much the end of our relationship. She*
> *announced that I was less spiritually evolved than she was and*
> *broke up. Since I had read the material on your website, I tried*
> *to tell her that she was having a separation hangover from orgasm.*
> *But she was buying none of that—although she did sort of see it*
> *after a few months had passed. I think orgasm's doing the oppo-*
> *site of what women want it to.*   *—Ken*

Not long after Anya and I faced the facts, I came upon a clue in black
and white that confirmed what we had learned the hard way. A Tantra
teacher in India wrote:

> [If a woman does not relax into a transcendental state during sex] she
> will have the nervous orgasm, which is short-lived and followed by
> dissatisfaction and exhaustion. This is often the cause of a woman's
> hysteria and depression.[19]

Not to mention that of her mate. So, if harmony in your relationship
is a goal, our experience suggests that women should not make the
same innocent error men have of believing tension-release orgasm is
the point of sex. Otherwise women could be setting up this familiar
scenario:

> This relationship was supposed to be different. We were bonded in
> spirit. But within six months we had fallen into the abyss of all that
> was unholy between man and woman. My physical and emotional
> health was severely depleted. Depression was a constant compan-
> ion. Our relationship was fragmented and wounded. How could I
> have experienced Divine Oneness and now feel such separation from

my husband? How could I endure the pain of not knowing how to close the enormous gap between us? What had happened during my marriage that warranted the comment from a new friend that I was the saddest looking woman she had ever seen? Before my marriage I was a professional educator, vibrantly alive. A year into it I felt drained of all but enough life force to survive.[20]

If you are still skeptical, get out a calendar and track it for yourself— both orgasms and pronounced mood swings over the following two to three weeks. If you are open-minded, you may see the connection between cause and effect for yourself.

If you are living with a partner, chances are your distress will be projected onto your partner. Ask for honest feedback. Watch for emotional separation between you ... whoever seems to cause it. When you learn to prevent this potent source of disharmony, you will find that all the other issues you thought were causing your discord mysteriously grow more manageable.

If women stop striving for genital orgasm, does this mean they give up all pleasure and return to their traditional role as asexual receptors of men's passion? Certainly not. It means that the satisfaction lovers have been looking for lies in a mutual experience in which both partners stop using each other for physical gratification and make nurturing each other their primary focus. As you will see, this causes a shift in body chemistry that heightens sexual responsiveness and makes all contact surprisingly enjoyable.

Incidentally, the first time I had orgasm during intercourse without striving for it at all was when I made love with a man who was a virgin. My attention was not on myself. I was focused entirely on making him feel safe and loved so the experience would always be a warm memory of loving intimacy. From that encounter onward I have been very orgasmic. And even though I now avoid orgasm because of the hangover, I still find that making my partner feel comfortable and adored is a sure turn-on for me.

People always think it's the seminal discharge that's undesirable, but it's actually the firing of the nervous system during sexual stimulation. And that applies to both men and women.

—Georg Feuerstein, Founder of the
Yoga Research and Education Center[21]

Orgasm is Orgasm

To be sure, that old biological itch is a formidable foe. Thwarted by the baffling alienation between the sexes, many of us have taken matters into our own hands. As you might expect, masturbation turned out to be another major blind spot, but let us start that part of the story, as I did, from a modern, mainstream vantage point.

If you have not checked out the magazines in the grocery line for a while, you might have missed the fact that masturbation is currently touted as a panacea, especially for women (*The Clitoral Truth: The Secret World at Your Fingertips* and *Sex for One: The Joy of Selfloving*), but also as therapy for couples (*Orgasms for Two: The Joy of Partner Sex*). Even Catholics are at last abandoning the nonsensical notion that masturbation is sinful, so good ole do-it-yourself sex appears to be the obvious solution ... for everyone ... for lots of things.

> Having sex is like playing bridge. If you don't have a good partner, you'd better have a good hand.

For example, it is a ready option when your post-orgasmic perception hangover makes your current partner sexually uninteresting. It also lets you find out how to have the most explosive orgasm possible, demonstrate for your lover, and provide for yourself when your lover lets you down. For many of us it is a sure-fire tranquilizer. And, of course, it is a way to relieve sexual frustration in between lovers.

Unfortunately all these rationalizations can lead you away from the goal of blissful harmony with another. The more you deplete yourself, the worse your partner will look. The more you chase explosive genital gratification, the more separation will unexpectedly erupt between you. And, perhaps most surprisingly of all, the more you masturbate, the more you decrease your power to attract a partner who is connecting with you for more than just sex. In short, whether you are pushed off a bridge or choose to jump, you are in for a rough landing. So regular masturbation is not the ideal means of managing sexual energy.

This, of course, does not imply that you should be afraid to touch your genitals, find out where things are, or be ashamed of what they are capable of doing. But continuing to research and practice what trips your trigger is of no benefit whatsoever if you wish to use sex to heal.

To tap your full potential you will have to move your prime focus from your genitals to your heart, so why not get started? The ultimate solution for sexual frustration is regular, nourishing exchanges with a lover, and, if you are without a partner, there are suggestions for the interim later in this chapter.

Meanwhile, I will touch on some aspects of masturbation that the grocery store magazines fail to mention, even though this discussion is a bit premature. As the next chapter will explain, intense genital stimulation causes neurochemical changes that promote addiction. So despite the initial relief a quick climax furnishes, it is junk food that leaves us feeling deprived at another level. We can swiftly become hooked on physical stimulation and conclude that orgasm, not union, is the point of having genitals.

Masturbation's aftereffects can leave us with a sense that something vital is lacking or that we are helpless to restore our sense of well-being. It may take a familiar form, such as discouragement, feeling painfully different from others, obstinacy, distrust, cynicism, baffling exhaustion, apathy, insomnia, and so forth. Few of us connect these feelings with frequent orgasm. Indeed, we may be certain that masturbation has had no ill effects on us. Yet, until we are clear of any addiction, we cannot accurately judge its effects.

When I went away to university I began masturbating about four times a day. My paranoia level grew noticeably. When someone once said, "Good Morning, Scott," I remember wondering, "What did he really mean by that?" Then I started using drugs a lot and dropped out after my first year. —Scott

---

Two of my friends who were addicted to masturbation were prescribed Prozac for inexplicable depression. (One ascribes his subsequent recovery to employing the suggestions in this book.) Depression furnishes fertile ground for other addictions, like marijuana and alcohol. So, as I cheerfully say to people, "Never feel bad about masturbating. It will make you feel bad enough." And it will do so whether or not you feel guilty about it. Guilt is just one version of the post-orgasm hangover. It may well take another form … like a certainty that you are being treated unfairly, cravings for unhealthy substances, or feeling unable to cope. Combine knowledge about this hangover with a new optimism about intimate relationships and you will find it relatively easy to abandon any further attempts at self-sufficiency and move purposefully toward union.

You asked why I have stopped masturbating. It is because I feel stronger and happier from day to day. I would not believe it if I did not experience it. There is also a laughing feeling in the stomach and throat all the time. Wonderful! My desire for social activities of any kind is much greater than one week or so after masturbating. I long for interaction with women, and it is just fine to exchange smiles here and there, or talk a little bit.

I remember that last year, before I tried to stop (or cut back...), I was constantly depressed. I did it nearly every other day and sometimes three or four times a day. It is rather hard to stop this addiction but THERE IS MUCH TO BE GAINED. In general: an awareness of the oneness of all.

Masturbation is a very powerful instrument to keep up the illusion of separation. This is the ultimate (spiritual) consequence of this practice.   —Karl

---

Incidentally, even as a tranquilizer, masturbation has hidden costs. The hangover from orgasm can impair judgment, causing a tendency to evade responsibility or jump nervously from one activity to the next in a hyperactive, but unproductive, manner. It can also promote irritability or a tendency to over-control. For example, I have noticed that frequent self-pleasuring tends to make some of my women friends especially brittle, particularly judgmental of men, and subject to intense mood swings. Behaviors like these alienate others more effectively than hairy palms. They are like ugly disguises that give us (and others) a very convincing, but false, impression of who we really are.

Masturbation also encourages fantasizing, and a compelling fantasy routine can entice us to remain in our own private world of self-gratification. Or, even when we connect with someone, we may find ourselves prisoner of our mental movie theater, unable to be fully present with our lover. While fantasy generally plays a big role in conventional sexual therapy, it is unnecessary with this approach. Orgasm is no longer the goal.

Increasing Sexual Magnetism

As the saying goes, like attracts like. So if you want to attract a relationship with the potential for balanced exchange (as opposed to a buddy bent on mutual over-stimulation), reach out and touch someone *else*. When we stop masturbating, our sexual magnetism increases. Some of the most seductive men on the planet hail from the West Indies. They take pride in using their sex appeal to draw women to them. They are successful in part because masturbation is not a big part of their culture. As a Jamaican friend once crooned when I asked him about masturbation in Jamaica, "Nooooooo . . . if you can't get a woman, dar is someting wrong wit you, mon." So, whether you are male or female, do not be afraid to charge up your battery. It will increase your charisma. You will make more of an effort to connect with others, and the more you do, the better you will feel.

Masturbation is a symptom of humankind's recurring sense of deprivation. As one friend explained: "Others are getting pleasure that I'm not, so I just look after myself." Unfortunately the attendant sense of emotional isolation too often creates a self-perpetuating cycle. The uneasiness that follows orgasm can cause us to hide in our caves—even if we think we really want a partner. As a German friend (who masturbated very frequently) put it:

> Thanks for your advice, but I cannot conjure a woman out of a cylinder like a rabbit. . . . I am still kind of wary thinking of women anyway. . . . Why should I give up the cozy privacy of my apartment for a strenuous woman??
>
> —Kai

His apartment was cramped, barren, and dominated by his computer with its various pornography subscriptions. A tomb provides refuge but has its limitations. The bottom line? The more we retreat into our own private world of self-gratification and self-pity, the less likely we are to attract a lover.

Union with another person offers the potential for satisfaction that managing our sexual energy alone cannot offer. At a deep level we all know this. Otherwise we do-it-yourself types would not even be reading a book on relationships. Our needs would be met. One man I spoke with had put it all together: "I know that when I have the uncontrollable need to masturbate, it's because I've passed up an opportunity to connect deeply with someone."

As we will see in a later chapter, medical research has confirmed that caring touch from another actually decreases the stress hormones our body pumps into us when, for example, we feed it angry, despairing messages. So if you have been a solo performer for a while, declare an intermission, and then try a duet. Meanwhile, find a massage therapist.

A break in the action can have its own rewards. When I visited Findhorn, a spiritual community in Scotland, returning visitors complained that the spiritual feelings they had experienced during earlier workshops would fade after they got home. A nineteen year-old Scot helped me see that part of the magic of Findhorn was probably the unaccustomed abstinence of its visitors. As my friend put it, he suffered from "Find-horniness" while he was there because he had to share a room for the week with another man whom he had never met. And he was busy with touchy-feely group activities each day. The combination took masturbation out of the picture for the week of the workshop. And he felt wonderful until soon after he got home, when his depressions and lack of focus mysteriously returned.

Q: How did Pinocchio discover he was made of wood?

A: His hand caught fire.

> *My abstinence continues (even without nocturnal semen losses, which surprises me). Now what I miss, more than wild sex, is tender moments with a woman. But I do not need a tenderness fix, because tenderness and intimacy are not addictive, while orgasm is. And you do not want to be tender with just anybody, because you need a person who really feels right.*
>
> *So now, after a couple weeks of cold turkey, I feel healed. For the first time in my life, I can wait. Does this explain what happened at last night's party? Two women insisted on giving me their phone numbers! In the past I always had to do the asking.*
>
> *—Antonio*

Meanwhile What Do I Do?

If you wish to attract a partner in order to try this new approach, you need the magnetic charge you would lose in masturbation. So for a month, at least, view masturbation as something you stop in order to increase your personal magnetism. Meanwhile, what do you do if you are bursting with life force energy, have met a potential partner you cannot yet snuggle with, or cannot sleep? Here are some techniques that others have found helpful, but keep in mind that they are temporary aids and cannot truly substitute for union:

- do movement work, martial arts, dancing, yoga, tai chi, or some other disciplined practice
- consciously circulate your sexual energy whenever you feel uncomfortably aroused. Close your eyes, tighten the muscles around your perineum, and draw the energy up your spine to the top of your head. Then imagine drawing it down the front of your body and storing it in your navel. (Some experts recommend inhaling as you draw the energy up your spine and exhaling as you draw the energy down the front of you. Others recommend inhaling as you draw it down through your heart, then tightening the muscles around your perineum and exhaling as the energy runs up your spine. Find out which works best for you.)
- do some spiritual work to open your heart and heal any lingering resentments
- exchange loving attention with the opposite sex even before your next partner appears. Start by giving. Invite a close friend of the opposite sex to take a walk. Give a foot massage with no strings attached. Hug a lot. Do a friend an unsolicited favor. Such actions not only guarantee that nice things come back to you, they also give you something productive to do with your pent-up sexual energy. As it flows outward in genuine service you will find your tensions are relieved while your heart stays open.

If you cannot completely stop having orgasms while on your own, do not get discouraged . . . find a partner. Except when in relationship, my partner never even attempted to give up masturbating (and depression was a constant problem). Other male friends report that if they do not relieve themselves, they tend to work themselves into exhaustion. When I was celibate for long periods of time, I sort of ran down. I tended to get colds, feel more anxious, accomplish less, and eventually have dream orgasms.

Even a rigorous spiritual practice is no guarantee of successful abstinence. One of my friends did Transcendental Meditation for years and was also without a partner. He noticed that his practice would take him to higher and higher states of bliss. After some weeks, however, his sexual energy would start to make him feel like he was going crazy. So he would masturbate and feel better for about a week.

The second week panic attacks would begin. One time he heard that radioactive waste was being disposed of in plastic and got the idea that his foam rubber pillow was going to cause cancer. He lay awake for nights. No logic would comfort him. He lived a nightmare. After a week of distress like this, he would begin to laugh at whatever had frightened him. Then he would feel better and better until the next cycle. For years he has avoided the only cure: union. He feels too fragile, too locked in his private world of meditation and masturbation, to enter into a relationship.

It is easy to conclude he has other issues, but I have seen radical improvements in levels of paranoia, confidence, and self-esteem in friends who have cut back on this seemingly harmless habit. So why not experiment with increasing your willpower? If you have an orgasm, how long is it until your next one in the form of a dream orgasm? You might use that interval as the basis of a schedule. Some Taoists propose ejaculation schedules for men that vary according to age and season of the year. And an Edgar Cayce reading recommended a hiatus of six to eight weeks.[22] In any case, here is a handy "rule of hand." If the sign below looks fuzzy to you, increase the intervals between self-pleasuring rituals.

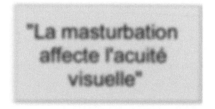

"La masturbation affecte l'acuité visuelle"

Translation:
Masturbation affects visual acuity
[Belgian humor from the Internet]

After all, what do you have to lose by changing your habits for a while and seeing how you feel? As one friend said, "It costs nothing, and at worst I pass up a few genital orgasms." If you do decide to cut back, make it easy for yourself—avoid dwelling on titillating sexual thoughts, stop mentally undressing others, and get rid of your vibrator. Resolutely steer clear of all romance novels, pornography, and movies with heavy sex. Such pastimes are powerful triggers and create cravings whether or not you masturbate all the way to orgasm.

And when you do get close to a partner, do not assume you will have more control if you masturbate first. Masturbation destabilizes you and lowers your sights. Try the slow, effortless approach recommended in Chapter 12 instead.

Now that you have some background in the unsuspected perils of the way we currently handle our innate sexual frustration, let us look again at humanity's circumstances from the evolutionary biology vantage point.

Summary

- ❧ The hangover caused by orgasm is present whether we masturbate or make love with someone.
- ❧ Despite its short-term payoff, orgasm can exacerbate neediness, emotional overreactions, and distancing behavior.
- ❧ Masturbation can increase feelings of self-pity, malaise, or irritability, fostering social isolation and addiction.
- ❧ Cutting back on masturbation increases sexual magnetism and decreases depression.

A Journalist, a Rabbi, and a Bard

Nature made it easy to get our engines going. Our sexual exuberance has all it needs to get us aroused, focused, mated and orgiastic. With the hypothalamus linking the endocrine system's hormones to the nervous system, and the limbic brain orchestrating the neurotransmitters of emotion, the sexual arc is figuratively and literally electrified. As the brain's pleasure centers light up, they bring not only joy to the moment of sex but also the appetite for more and more sex. The all-time best aphrodisiac for sex remains sex itself. The more we have it the more we want it. It is the ultimate addiction.

—Joann Ellison Rodgers, *SEX: A Natural History*

Most of a person's drives are his biological impulses, which seek to be gratified. If you find yourself being attracted to do something, pause and lean a bit toward not doing it. That way you will maintain an even balance.

—Rabbi of Rizhin, nineteenth-century Chassidic Sage

Th'expense of spirit in a waste of shame
Is lust in action; and, till action, lust
Is perjured, murd'rous, bloody, full of blame,
Savage, extreme, rude, cruel, not to trust;

Enjoyed no sooner but despised straight;
Past reason hunted, and no sooner had,
Past reason hated as a swallowed bait
On purpose laid to make the taker mad;

Mad in pursuit, and in possession so;
Had, having, and in quest to have, extreme;
A bliss in proof, and proved, a very woe,
Before, a joy proposed; behind, a dream.

All this the world well knows, yet none knows well
To shun the heaven that leads men to this hell.

—William Shakespeare, *Sonnet 129*

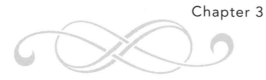

Chapter 3

Biology Has Plans for Your Love Life

As mentioned in the Introduction, biology spurs us to connect with or abandon partners to further *its* goals, even at the expense of our relationships. I mentioned that women are more likely to be unfaithful during their most fertile days of the month.[23] And even when infidelity is not an issue, their biological programming can cause them to make superficial choices.

> *Being a woman who is extremely sensitive to my ovulation cycle, I can ATTEST that I am personally vulnerable to "good DNA subjects" (i.e., good-looking men) when I'm fertile. This tendency is totally gone at every other time of the month. When my biological process is at bay, I relate with people on a more intellectual, or culturally relevant, level. It's quite bizarre. —Jasmine*

Women also tend to choose mates based largely on body odor (pheromones). The scents they are drawn to correlate with genetic advantages for potential offspring rather than long-term compatibility. Specifically, the more varied our genetic immunity, the more robust we are. So a woman is drawn to a partner whose aroma indicates genetic immunity that is diverse from her own.[24] And, as stated in the Introduction, women also orgasm more frequently with genetically sound specimens, and female orgasm during intercourse improves the chance of conception by increasing semen retention. So orgasm, in women, as in men, turns out to be more about genetic strategy than healthy companionship or even physical gratification.

Similarly, male biology zombies, whatever their age, find themselves helplessly attracted to women who look like they could make a lot of babies, i.e., *young* women. This occurs even when men consciously do not wish to be fathers, and would genuinely find the companionship of a peer more comforting. We judge men to be emotionally shallow while biology bewitches them, but the point is that genetic greediness, for all of us, is so predictable that we are naïve to mistake it for *our* will.

Absence Makes the Sperm Count Higher
The more time couples spend together between ejaculations, the fewer sperm the man delivers during conventional intercourse. That is, males apparently perceive sperm competition in mates who have been out of sight, and ejaculate as many as four times more sperm to improve their chances of fathering offspring. No one knows how this mechanism works, but biology can clearly manipulate our behavior without our conscious participation.[25]

When given free rein, our biological programming will blithely imperil an existing relationship in favor of an additional, or improved, fertilization opportunity. Indeed, most men (and many women) can attest to the power of the Coolidge Effect, which got its name many years ago when President Coolidge and his wife were touring a farm. While the President was elsewhere, the farmer proudly showed Mrs. Coolidge a rooster that "could copulate with hens all day long, day after day."

Mrs. Coolidge coyly suggested he tell that to Mr. Coolidge. The farmer did. The President thought for a moment and then inquired, "With the same hen?"

"No, sir," replied the farmer.

"Tell that to Mrs. Coolidge," retorted the President.

So how does biology persuade us to meet its agenda at the expense of our relationships? It simply turns up the volume in our primitive brain (limbic system) so loud that it drowns out conflicting signals, particularly the ones warning us that we will soon regret our actions.

A Neurochemical Arsenal

Perhaps you have had this experience: you are cheerfully sauntering along when suddenly . . . smack! Hit by an arrow . . . or was it a tank? Oh my God! Has anyone ever felt like you are now feeling? How does old Cupid do it? Well, he dips that arrow in a lot of neurochemicals that evoke powerful responses in your primitive brain. One of them is PEA, a neurochemical so stimulating that lab mice injected with it bounce around like popping corn. Another is adrenaline, which gets your heart racing. A third is dopamine, also known as the master molecule of addiction. And all of this drama is being played out in your brain, not your genitals.

Why the overkill? Why can't falling in love be as romantic as a valentine, and as cuddly as a down comforter?

Evolutionary biologists would say it is because Cupid's real name is Gene. That is, the purpose behind this powerful instinctual response is not love, but reproduction. Your genes, the greedy little critters, will go to any lengths to get you to replicate more of them. Their goal is simple: immortality. So far, at least, they have succeeded. With every baby we still replicate some of the same genes that were present in the planet's earliest life forms.

"Is it true, Dad, that in some parts of Africa a man doesn't know his wife until he marries her?"

"Son, that happens in every country."

Humankind sometimes flatters itself that evolution's goal has been to design a perfect physical organism—us. In actuality, our genes measure their success by quantity (the more the better) and variety. Variety allows them to meet changing environmental conditions and still keep the production lines rolling. Quality is not their goal, except to the extent it makes possible greater quantity.

Obviously humanity has been successful in evolutionary terms. Indeed, with population levels mushrooming out of control, we may soon prove too successful. We owe much of this dubious accomplishment to our burning desire to have sex. Our design is programmed with many inducements to keep us reproducing at top speed, especially during the years when we are likely to produce the soundest physical specimens.

Dopamine, a Debatable Friend

The most obvious and easily manipulated stimulus is the pleasure/reward center deep within our primitive brain. This structure has been around for millions of years and has not changed much. It is present in all mammals, and it is why rats and humans can get hooked on the same drugs.

The reward center is a group of nerve cells that are usually activated when we engage in activities or behaviors that once increased our ancestors' chances of survival (and reproduction). We receive rewards for:

- *eating high-calorie foods* because the best way nomadic ancestors could store food was as fat;
- *taking risks* and *winning* because bold, aggressive lovers were more likely to pass on their genes; and, above all,
- *having sex,* even when a harsh existence did not leave our ancestors with much opportunity for hanky-panky, or energy/resources for raising offspring.

As scientists Burnham and Phelan, the authors of *Mean Genes, From Sex to Money to Food, Taming our Primal Instincts,*[26] point out, such activities now create more havoc than good. For example,

- High-calorie foods are too plentiful for many of us, but we continue to receive our biological reward for ordering extra fries. This pat on the back for impulsive consuming, rather than prudence, also leads some of us to run up nasty credit card debts.
- The reward for taking risks/winning sometimes proves equally treacherous. We develop gambling addictions or obsessions for extreme sports/reckless activities because they offer such a buzz. And the lust to win (elections, more money, lofty titles) ensures that we frequently compromise our principles or even commit crimes.
- Sexual stimulation is readily available these days, and our built-in compulsion to orgasm frequently leads to rash, aggressive, or just plain stupid sexual behavior.

The reward center's cells are activated by a neurochemical called dopamine. It ignites this section of the primitive brain with intense *anticipation* of pleasure. Its message is, "This is it! Do not miss your chance! Go for it, whatever you have to do to get it!" In fact, the dopamine reward is so compelling that in an experiment where rats could push a lever to stimulate the portion of their brains on which it acts, they "blissed" themselves till they dropped, without pausing to eat or investigate sexually receptive partners.[27] Not surprisingly, dopamine surges are behind all addictions.

When sex evaporated from my marriage bed, I thought that what had been missing was passion. In fact, I prayed for the return of what I called "passion" in my life. It surfaced in the form of a red-haired Scorpio who looked excellent in hot pants. At some point during the stormy ride that followed, I stumbled upon a dictionary definition of passion. "Any intense emotion," *it said,* "such as the sufferings of Jesus upon the cross." *Sure enough I had found passion, all right. Brief as it was, our relationship made crucifixion look kind of appealing. I now realize that what I really want is love ... not suffering.*   —*Christopher*

Dopamine, like all neurochemicals, defies simple categorization as good or bad. Each neurochemical has multiple roles in the body. The complexity of the interactions of related neurochemicals boggles the mind and is far from completely mapped out. Still, it is fascinating to hypothesize about the implications of the recent flood of scientific evidence on how neurochemicals interact with our emotions and behavior.

Because of its role in addiction, dopamine has been studied extensively. At ideal levels it plays a vital role in feelings of cheerful anticipation, healthy appetite, and may also be connected with motivating us to make rewarding choices. At higher levels, though, it is behind cravings, uncontrolled behavior, unrealistic thinking, and thrill-seeking. Because of dopamine, "drugs of abuse produce the same exhilaration, excessive energy, sleeplessness, and loss of appetite that are characteristic of individuals who report being 'in love.'"[28] Excess dopamine has been implicated in sexual fetishes as well.[29] And high levels are also found in the brains of schizophrenics, who, instead of being cheerful, are often delusional, agitated, and irritable.[30]

Dopamine's effect on libido accounts for claims like this one from a sales site on the Internet:

WARNING, this dopamine fire formula can turn men and women to sexual mania. We are not responsible for your sexual manic behaviors after taking this package.

As scientists Quartz and Sejnowski put it, "Although Mae West once said that too much of a good thing is wonderful, dopamine is different."[31] Too much dopamine transforms healthy anticipation into an aching craving with the power to subvert our wills, make us anxious, give us a false sense of invincibility, or turn us into addicts—all with no lasting satisfaction or genuine contribution to our well-being.

Dopamine, the craving neurochemical, is the driving force behind sex. Foreplay (anticipation) leads to a rise in dopamine until the point of orgasm with its own burst of pleasure neurochemicals. Although anticipation of orgasm is intensely compelling thanks to dopamine, the more satisfying reward of orgasm is probably a blend of natural opiates (endorphins), which may be enhanced by the effects of oxytocin, a neurochemical associated with open-hearted feelings and a desire to bond.

These other, more beneficial neurochemical rewards (endorphins and oxytocin) are not dependent upon a fiery dopamine anticipation phase—as long-term meditators and those who engage in ecstatic prayer, could tell you. That is, blissful satisfaction is possible *without* excess dopamine in the picture. Biology has manipulated us into linking the two, thereby creating the ultimate addiction.

Do We Want to Follow Biology's Script for Our Love Lives?

We all like to think that we can sustain both our genes' heady reward for fertilization behavior and romance indefinitely in the same relationship. Yet relationships tend to blossom until some point after sex enters the picture. Different couples reach this point of diminishing returns at different times, but this U-turn is so universal that popular wisdom predicts the honeymoon period of a marriage will last less than one year. And, as we will see in Chapter 6, a recent Ohio State University study of hundreds of couples bears this out.[32] Basically we are designed to binge on sex until we reach a point of excess, and then we are repelled from further indulgence, at least temporarily. This feast-or-famine pattern harms our relationships.

It may still not be obvious to you how both of you having as many orgasms as possible could lead to disharmony, but suppose a drug dealer intentionally seduced you with free cocaine until you were hooked. On one hand, you would light up with anticipated pleasure whenever you saw him coming. At another level, however, you would resent him because of the control he exerts over your happiness due to your dependency.

> "Honey, when we were together, you always said you'd die for me. Now that we're divorced, don't you think it's time you kept your promise?"

Also, think how distressed you would feel if he did not show up with the drug when you were counting on it. And what if he did not give you any just because you did little but get high all the time and had nothing to give in return? How cruel, right? The intensity of your feelings would reflect your degree of neediness, rather than the depth of your emotional connection. You would not be concerned with his well-being at all.

It is normal to feel mistreated if we cannot get our fix, whether it comes from sex or elsewhere. But we feel equally resentful if someone uses us as a fix when addiction has eroded his/her capacity to care genuinely about us. No wonder we often want to run away, seek comfort from someone else, or change partners because we sense something unhealthy is going on. And we never see that delivering great sex is helping to create relationship dysfunction.

Our neurochemistry tells us a big lie: that the intensity of our cravings is a measure of the value of the reward that lies around the corner. We were bred to find sexual cravings so delicious that we would give no thought to the consequences of yielding to them, whether those consequences are unwanted

> If love is blind, why is lingerie so popular?
>
> —George Carlin

pregnancy or merely an uncomfortable hangover period that causes relationship deterioration. In truth, the cure for our ills is *not* more dopamine and more dependency, or a better orgasm supply (through infidelity, casual sex, or coercing our partner in some way).

The cure is to heal ourselves of our dependency while carefully preserving the advantages of intimate union: better health, personal growth, inner equilibrium, and a sense that all is right with the world. As we shed our need to manipulate others to meet our fervent desires, right and wrong are obvious again. Our self-image improves. We see how powerful we are and can view our past mistakes with greater compassion. When free of the invisible cords of this addiction, we recognize how tightly it bound us and how high were its costs. We also see that it is possible to feel sparklingly alive and sexy without the rushes of excitement associated with excess dopamine.

Author Gilles Marin contrasts appetite, which is a healthy, with craving. A craving is always for something we should avoid because if we obtain it, we will only desire more of it. In effect, we reinforce our neediness.

> Lust is sexual craving. It is born out of the inability to satisfy our sexuality. . . . We try over and over again, often with different partners, with the sad result that every unsuccessful attempt builds a potential of failure that inevitably will end up in depression. A lack of knowing better in matters of sexual satisfaction, and an overload of pent-up energy, are usually the different factors that lead to lust. Yielding to sexual cravings leads rapidly to a huge loss of vital energy and is destructive to oneself and others.[33]

Prolactin —
The Lights-Out Signal?

I am not aware of any research done directly on the neurochemistry behind the emotional distance between lovers after sex. But my partner did track down some recent research that suggests prolactin may be part of the reason for it.

At climax, dopamine begins to shut down. Its mission, inciting a fertilization attempt, has been accomplished. One of the reasons we have been having so much fun is that dopamine, in addition to making us crave orgasm, has been serving as a brake on another neurochemical called prolactin. Prolactin, as its name suggests, was once thought to confine its effects to promoting lactation in mothers. But according to recent research, it also plays a rather unwelcome role in the sex lives of both genders.

When prolactin rises after orgasm it acts as a sexual satiation mechanism. It is probably behind the post-ejaculation roll over and snore phenomenon. No one knows how long its influence typically lingers. However, mating triggered surges in prolactin levels for at least three days in rats.[34] It is likely that the duration and severity of prolactin's effects vary considerably from person to person depending upon body chemistry and state of mind. Multi-orgasmic people, for example, appear to be able to keep going *because* prolactin levels do not rise after their initial orgasms.[35]

In any event, consistently high prolactin levels can cause sexual dysfunction and menstrual irregularities, make us feel depressed, and even decrease bone density.[36] Some have surmised that, because prolactin levels tend to rise with age, prolactin is part of nature's plan to get us out of the way of subsequent generations.

The good news is that any of us can make love indefinitely without triggering this damper, as long as we do not climax. Could this be why various ancient sacred sex traditions advised avoiding orgasm to improve health and increase longevity?

As we were falling asleep after making love, I noticed that my lover still had a strong erection. We had just started experimenting with avoiding orgasm during sex, so I asked him, "Isn't that making you uncomfortable?" I could hear a big smile in his voice as he replied, "No, I love it!" And when we woke up during the night, I found out why. . . . —Kaiya

No! No! A Thousand Times No!

While the hormones of almost all other mammals force them to observe breaks in sexual activity until females are in heat again, humans can mate anytime. We can also force our way around our prolactin-induced slumps . . . in the short run. How? By driving up our dopamine levels again, whatever it takes. In other words, clever primates that we are, we do not wait for our sexual appetite to return naturally.

Our hunger for a dopamine surge throws us into an addictive cycle. Genuine desire for closer union may no longer be our primary motivation for making love, because our body is now simply trying to avoid the pain of withdrawal brought on by over-stimulation. In effect, we may use our partner to self-medicate. We want more and hotter sex, too, because our pleasure nerves grow less and less responsive, as I will explain in a moment.

Sometimes no partner is available, or our partner looks unappealing because we are projecting the uneasiness of our neurochemical hangover onto him/her. So we may opt for frequent masturbation, or hijack the pleasure/reward mechanism with unhealthy activities that also raise dopamine levels: alcohol, gambling, recreational drugs, reckless spending, or overeating. Sound familiar?

In the long run, most of us would have been better off waiting out the slump like our less-calculating mammalian cousins.

Clearly we are designed to find fertilization behavior so compelling that we need some sort of regulation. Otherwise, like the rats mentioned above, we would tend to ignore vital aspects of our well-being to pursue orgasm (or its dopamine-elevating substitutes). The prolactin-induced slump is, of course, a regulatory mechanism. For example, nursing mothers, with high levels of prolactin, are notorious for their lack of interest in sex. When? Right at the time that their infants—our genes' next wave of reproduction machines—critically need their full attention.

Nor is prolactin the only disciplinarian. Our pleasure nerve cells also attempt to restore us to equilibrium. In response to over-stimulation by dopamine, some the tiny dopamine receptors on our cells temporarily shut down. And until these receptors reawaken, normal

On the Effects of Prolactin: Paul returns from a doctor's visit having learned that he has only twenty-four hours to live. Wiping away his wife's tears, he asks to make love. Of course she agrees. Six hours later, Paul goes to her, "Maybe we could make love again?" They make love. Later, Paul is getting into bed, "Honey? Please? Just one more time before I die." She agrees. Four hours later he taps his wife on the shoulder. "Honey, could we . . . ?" She sits up abruptly, turns and says, "Listen, Paul, I have to get up in the morning. You don't."

amounts of dopamine, which are crucial to our ideal sense of cheerful anticipation about life, will not trigger the usual response. Sex feels different. This protective down-regulation mechanism also occurs with recreational drug use and accounts for the crash after using cocaine, amphetamines, ecstasy, and so forth.

As with surging prolactin, the shutdown of dopamine receptors can have various unpleasant side effects ranging from anxiety and irritability to severe depression. At a neurochemical level the joy has literally gone out of our lives. And the harder we try to force a renewed sense of well-being with more dopamine (sex, drugs, food, watching sports or movies, surfing the Internet), the more likely our nerve cells will down-regulate further to try to return us to a natural, healthy equilibrium.

In short, the post-orgasmic drop in dopamine and rise in prolactin deliver a powerful one-two punch that can temporarily decrease our sense of well-being. And constant efforts to get around it can actually ensure chronic uneasiness or escapism, except for brief, forced bursts of excess dopamine.

The Great Awakening: Relationship Disharmony

Like starting and stopping in city traffic, biology's strategy for regulating our sexual behavior is very hard on our relationships. In fact, things can get really ugly while we are out of sorts. Here is an extreme example. A friend of mine had severe urinary tract infection during the months following her marriage. She and her husband both liked sex, and by the time she was in severe pain, urinating blood, her husband was so hooked on orgasm that he informed her he was demanding his marital rights at least three times a week regardless of her condition. When focused on attaining such an intense reward, our judgment is often impaired.

A determination to feel good again can make us unbearably insistent that others meet our temporarily exaggerated needs, whether we are demanding more sex or someone to clean out the garage. Our partner will understandably grow defensive. Neediness and

"Aw c'mon. Who the @#$% is going to find out?"
—Bill Clinton, 1999

defensiveness effectively stop the production of the neurochemical that gives us the urge to bond with each other. Then we may withhold much-needed affection, take remarks the wrong way, be less generous, see each other's faults in an exaggerated manner, and perhaps find each other less attractive.

Such neurochemical shifts even make some of us violent.

> Chinese medicine long ago observed that vicious crimes are often committed soon after seminal loss. Courage is usually at low ebb after ejaculation. One scares easily and reacts violently.[37]

Women under biology's spell are equally powerfully programmed to ignore the welfare of others. They frequently choose to produce babies, regardless of the circumstances, and have them supported at another's expense. Two friends come to mind who both went bankrupt because their lovers got pregnant and insisted on having children against the men's advice—even though the relationships were not stable, there was severe economic hardship, the women were not "right-to-lifers," and in one case the woman had assured her long-term partner that a condom was unnecessary because she could not become pregnant. Pushing men into fatherhood is, like sexual aggression, fundamentally forgivable because the perpetrators are under biological hypnosis. At another level, however, such behaviors are appalling. Tragically, the resulting wariness between the sexes keeps us from tapping the deeper rewards of union.

At any rate, perhaps you are beginning to see how your relationship can feel like an emotional roller coaster ride of intense highs and lows while biology pulls your strings. After an initial neurochemical frenzy of attraction, partners seldom find that their desire and satiation cycles synchronize well. And our naive attempts to soothe ourselves with more pleasure make us selfish or make us feel like martyrs, however healthy and loving our true nature.

> *Romantic attraction is both a positive and negative emotion. It has stimulated the world's greatest poetry and many of our happiest moments. But it can also be the basis of stalkers, homicides, clinical depression and suicide. —Helen Fisher, anthropologist*

Biology leaves us waffling between inflated expectations, inspired by biology's initial fertilization strategy, and cynical pessimism, brought on by our body's self-regulation efforts. Over time these exaggerated reactions cause hurt feelings, emotional distance, and unhappy relationships. And the repercussions extend beyond infidelity and divorce. As we will see, our relationship can actually become a threat to our health instead of enhancing our well-being.

Meanwhile, our genes sail through generation after generation untroubled by our distress because serial relationships, and even infidelity, serve the other governing principle of genetic strategy: increasing the number of genetic combinations. However, we as individuals suffer enormously. And we remain at biology's mercy until we begin to make the connection between that great sex we had last week and the disharmony we are experiencing this week.

Gene Wars
Biology has the sexes bickering with each other all the way down to their genes. For example, a mother's genetic immortality is best served by smaller offspring; otherwise she will be less likely to survive to produce more progeny. But large offspring have a better chance of surviving to pass on their own genes. So, according to the theory of David Haig of Harvard University, paternal genes favoring fetal growth war with maternal genes that limit growth.

WANTED: Meaningful Overnight Relationship

Over time, the dopamine/prolactin hangover can cause subconscious uneasiness between you and *every* lover. It remains in your psyche like a rusty but fully operational bear trap, even when you avoid the behavior that forces too much stimulation. This is because your amygdala, the part of your primitive brain that archives emotional memories, has carefully recorded that your dopamine highs are followed by distress. Its job is to protect you against repeating past errors. So until you take the time to consciously lay down a new conditioned response to intimacy, it faithfully sends you a gut feeling of uneasiness when you get close to anything it has associated with painful past events.

This protective portion of the primitive brain is extremely short-sighted. It does not realize that fallout from over-stimulation is the source of your distress. After all, orgasm felt great. Instead, it registers the problem as your relationship, because that is where the problems usually show up. Its motto is: sex is good—relationships are dangerous. It issues its warnings chemically, and so quickly that they can activate your body's defense reactions before your neo-cortex (the part of your brain that analyzes logically) even has a chance to evaluate your circumstances.[38]

So your amygdala may send you bail-out messages immediately after your first orgasm with a new partner. Or it may kick on when you even approach anyone with whom you could form a real relationship. While the amygdala is guarding you from ongoing intimacy, stable, generous partners just will not turn you on. And you will not even bother to question your verdict. "Oh, there was no spark between us."

If you want a committed lover, look in a mental institution.

Mysteriously, however, you will find unavailable, incompatible partners (those with *Exit* signs flashing behind their heads) ever so attractive. I call this the *Romance Junkie Syndrome,* and you can determine whether you are one in the material following this chapter. If you have become a Romance Junkie, you can thank your amygdala for your fixation on non-relationships.

Another Noble Experiment

All this brain chemistry led me to one vital insight. To protect our relationship, my partner and I would have to learn to make love differently, limiting the production of dopamine to comfortable levels and avoiding orgasm with its prolactin-induced slump. Years of experience had confirmed that each orgasm sets off another cycle of highs and lows. That temporarily stops all progress toward teaching our bodies to produce the alternative, more balanced combination of feel-good neurochemicals I will talk about in the next chapter.

Some gains from the avoid-orgasm approach were already obvious to me. I had once had to take antibiotics almost every time I made love just to avoid urinary tract infection. I have not used them in more than ten years with this method. And a friend of mine with genital herpes who also experimented with this approach noticed that outbreaks did not occur except when he wandered back into a search for passion. I wanted to see what other miracles lay ahead. I proposed that we try the *Exchanges,* the series of activities in Chapter 12 designed to help couples lay down a new response to sexual arousal.

For Will, however, this was all uncharted territory. Here is his account of his initial experience, written after about ten months:

> When I agreed to try the *Exchanges,* I had my reservations. Number one, I'd never been able to sleep comfortably through the night with anyone. Number two, I wasn't thrilled about making love according to some recipe that sounded like *it* would tell *me* when I could have intercourse. Three, I didn't know Marnia *that way,* and it felt weird to start on a program that envisioned making love some weeks down the road. Four, I liked masturbating as much as anyone (about three or four times a week), and I knew I'd have to give up ejaculation.
>
> I had read her material, though, and it perfectly described the roller coaster of my previous relationships. Finally, I understood why I'd always pulled away to find my own "space," or gotten into pointless arguments with my lovers. I sensed that this approach to sex might be the answer. A few months earlier I had broken up again with the mother of my son, with whom I'd had a painful, on-and-off-again relationship. I'd started drinking immediately after we got together the first time, fifteen years earlier.
>
> By the time I started the *Exchanges,* my life was a mess. I was in financial ruin and my drinking had increased to the point where I knew I was an alcoholic. I was spiraling downward and I didn't know how to get myself back up. I decided it was worth a try.
>
> Some effects of the *Exchanges* were surprisingly rapid. After only three days I felt more comfortable and relaxed in my body. Kissing started to feel like a whole different experience—like my first kisses many years earlier. Outcome-based sex fell away. And my focus on my genitals started to shift to more of a focus on sharing.

Other changes followed. The problem of being able to sleep with someone disappeared, though the first few nights were challenging. Now I love holding her if I awaken in the night before we fall back asleep.

The addiction took longer to address—in part because I tried to hide it while I struggled to stop on my own ... repeatedly ... and with no success. When it came out in the open I was sure she would leave ... but she didn't. Instead we became partners in addressing it. It has been more than six months since I've had any alcohol, and I haven't had cravings or withdrawal symptoms. Occasionally I've had some thoughts about drinking ... always following overheating her or myself. Previously, I used alcohol to escape from the pain of relationship. But with this approach the relationship has been a source of inspiration and strength.

I haven't ejaculated at all since the relationship began ten months ago, and the desire to have orgasm isn't really present—though I'm sure I could if I wanted to. There have been no ill effects from not ejaculating. I've had only one experience of genital discomfort, which occurred when she overheated me with classic foreplay.

The biggest difference between this relationship and my others is that we feel like teenagers, even though we're in our forties. We spend an hour or more kissing most days and make love frequently. The energy's been like that between us from the beginning—except for a few detours into "relationship hell," brought on by too much passion, which led to her climaxing. They've convinced me that if we were engaging in conventional sex, my relationship with her would be as dismal as any of my past relationships.

I've seen big changes in other aspects of my life, too. My finances are sorting themselves out, and my professional life is expanding in directions I'd always wanted it to—but was unable to take it before. The opportunities continue to flow to me effortlessly and work out great. I have a lot more confidence in myself. I'm calm and focused. And I'm now comfortable with being in a partnership instead of seeing myself as a separate entity that happens to be involved with someone at the same time. I'm much more optimistic about relationships.

It was apparent that we were better off without classic orgasm. Yet, as you will see in the next chapter, there was more to eluding Cupid's/Gene's arrows than simply skipping the "Big O."

Summary

- Most of us release prolactin after each orgasm. It lowers libido and can cause depression.
- Too much of the neurochemical dopamine, associated with intense desire and recklessness, sets off a subsequent cycle of anxiety or craving, as our nerve cells seek to protect themselves against further over-stimulation.
- When our subconscious registers that sexual intimacy creates problems, it is more likely to perceive ongoing intimacy as the culprit than to perceive over-stimulation as the cause. This misperception occurs because the fallout from our hangover so often shows up as disharmony in our relationships.
- To us it seems like the actual sex was great, while our relationship is now excruciating. Obvious but mistaken solution? Grab the sex, avoid ongoing intimacy, and move on.
- Unfortunately, grabbing for more fiery neurochemistry endangers our well-being because it sets us on an addictive quest that will yield less satisfaction over time.

Are You a Romance Junkie?

Do you find yourself consistently choosing partners

- whom you find when you (or they) are far away from home?
- who dumped you abruptly before?
- whom you can only see for brief encounters due to their (or your) professional or parental commitments?
- who are married to others?
- who have a long history of brief affairs?

Do you fall in love with such partners and have intense romantic encounters?

If you answer yes to these two questions, you are likely to be a Romance Junkie. You have already figured out that sex with your heart open is an experience far superior to just having sex. But your subconscious is still fearful of ongoing intimacy because of the associated emotional chaos.

Your solution is to predetermine an escape route that your subconscious believes will allow you to elude the inevitable fallout. And so you are fearless during the encounter and easily open your heart. Indeed, a Romance Junkie can have orgasms that feel like profound spiritual experiences and are as compelling as mainlining heroin. They have all the drawbacks, too:

- They create hangovers, even if your subconscious does not register the cause-and-effect link. Though your mystical encounter may remain untarnished in your mind, your life will reflect back to you your subsequent sense of uneasiness. Frequently it shows up in the form of disappointment, illness, depression, financial woes, etc.
- You cannot master sexual self-control in fleeting, intense encounters. First, you have not built up the balance and inner strength that makes control a real possibility, and second, the temptation to go for orgasm is usually overpowering when you are not likely to see each other again or any time soon.
- And, as a Romance Junkie, you are hooked on non-relationships. In fact, you cannot get your accustomed high in a relationship with possible commitment looming.

It may take time, but being a Romance Junkie gradually leads to stagnation. You are always planning your escape or feeling victimized by departing lovers. Your will is actually imprisoned by your defenses. And, like any other addict, you are not inclined to go through a dissatisfying withdrawal period in favor of forming real relationships. Why? Because they will not meet your craving for the "great sex" you are hooked on. To feel those highs again, you must learn to open your heart in situations where commitment is a real possibility. That will take some time and mutual healing.

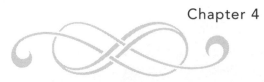

Chapter 4

A Change
of Heart

AS YOU CAN SEE FROM THE LAST CHAPTER, BIOLOGY continually sows the seeds of separation in our relationships in its drive to meet its goals. In effect, it tells us to do it, and then to *quit* doing it. Dopamine rushes of intense anticipation set off mini manic-depressive cycles, which are probably more pronounced due to the effects of prolactin (the sexual satiation neurochemical). These mood swings can cause us to see our partners through dark-colored glasses, creating agitation and emotional friction.

Even worse, we feel betrayed. The world becomes a frightening place when relationships or behaviors that *feel* like they will powerfully benefit us so often lead instead to fleeting gratification . . . and painful long-term repercussions. Over the years, as we are repeatedly battered by this fertilization-reward mechanism, we end up anxious or angry, emotionally isolated, and less and less fulfilled.

There is a way around this problem, but not while too much dopamine with its spellbinding fire and distressing hangover is at work in our brains. We must elude Cupid's/Gene's arrow. We are equipped

> "I am" is reportedly the shortest sentence in the English language. Could it be that "I do" is the longest sentence?
> —George Carlin

to do this if we so choose. We can protect ourselves by learning to sustain the body chemistry for emotional bonding and unconditional love. The prime player is a hormone called oxytocin. Both nursing mothers and newborns normally produce high levels of it. It permanently rearranges their brain structures by establishing new connections. Hence the deep, lifelong bond between care-giving parents and their children.

Biology's use for this bonding chemistry is, of course, strictly related to procreation. Lovers, too, are flooded with oxytocin and create bonding neural configurations—because biology wants us to stick around long enough to get the kids off to a good start.[39] But then it hopes we will move on to new genetic opportunities. Its strategy often succeeds because the addictive, dopamine-based highs of conventional sex fade, leaving one or both partners dissatisfied. Their brains then establish neural patterns of defensiveness that gradually, or rapidly, override the loving configuration.

We are not prisoners of this blueprint. And the loophole in biology's plan is our capacity for deep emotional bonding and altruism. We have only to protect and strengthen these natural ties by using our bodies and relationships differently. We can do that by consciously encouraging the production of oxytocin—and *must* do so if we wish to stay in love. We simply nurture each other without selfish motive instead of using each other as biology intended. The gains from this simple shift are not limited to relationship harmony. They include improved health and longer lives as well.

If we can learn to maintain the ideal levels of dopamine, oxytocin, and other pleasure neurochemicals (by making equilibrium our goal), we can enjoy ongoing sexual intimacy without hangovers. Indeed, scientific research and experience suggest that the right combination of dopamine and oxytocin can turn a neutral sexual experience into a strongly positive and reinforced one that lasts.[40]

Such an approach may be unfamiliar to us today but it is hardly new. Thousands of years ago the Taoists recorded that the less passionate path of intercourse can lead to an ecstatic relaxation orgasm rather than a forced tension-and-release orgasm. Whether or not you experience a total relaxation orgasm with this gentler approach, you will relish your enhanced inner balance. A profound sense of well-being increases as you move away from the degenerating cycle of highs and lows. And, as your amygdala (emotional memory bank) relaxes its subconscious guard, your heart opens even further.

Love is when you go out to eat and give somebody most of your french fries without making them give you any of theirs.

—*Chrissy, age 6*

A Closer Look at Oxytocin

Oxytocin is the caring hormone. It has also been called the cuddle hormone, the love hormone, and the open-heart hormone. Without it, lab animals showed less concern for others and increased aggression. So if you have ever watched a lover grow insensitive or move into a "sex is just sex and you need to give it to me" mindset or an "I don't care how much you're suffering, there will be no sex for you" mindset, you can bet your beloved is just experiencing a drop in oxytocin. It is time to change your lovemaking habits.

Scientists only recently uncovered this nurturing feature of oxytocin. Previously they believed that it confined its effects to labor contractions and milk ejection. Oxytocin was therefore wrongly assumed to have no appreciable effects on men. Actually its role in romantic bonding is quite dramatic for both sexes. Without it we could not fall in love.

And that is only the half of it. Oxytocin exerts tremendous additional influences on the brain and behavior that are just coming to light. For example, it increases the sexual receptivity of females[41] and aids in erection of the penis. In other words, it gives intimacy its stardust.

It also increases the attraction between partners, but not between unfamiliar potential mates.[42] So it can make your lover look delicious without increasing your sexual attraction to strangers. It is thus far different from the often rather blind, purely sexual hunger that excess dopamine ignites.

In short, if we want the advantages of monogamy (which are many, as we will see), then we must learn

Men and women are different in the morning. We men wake up aroused. We can't help it. We just wake up and we want you. And the women are thinking, 'How can he want me the way I look in the morning?' It's because we can't see you. We have no blood anywhere near our optic nerve.
—Andy Rooney

to keep our oxytocin levels up. Sustained oxytocin levels are the antidote to our preprogrammed uneasiness and four-year itch. (Four years
is about how long researchers estimate we are designed to stay together,
according to Rutgers anthropologist Helen Fisher, Ph.D.)

As we fall in love we are obviously producing a lot of oxytocin. So
why is this wonder hormone not strong enough to withstand the post-
orgasmic dopamine-induced prolactin slump? The short answer is
that it often is . . . for a time. That is why new couples think I am
crazy to suggest that their seemingly solid, obviously loving, and very
sexual relationships are in jeopardy if they do not change the way they
make love.

Not surprisingly, humanity's false confidence is neurochemically
induced. Oxytocin levels usually rise briefly at the moment of orgasm,
so most of us assume sex is the most powerful glue there is. Indeed,
we instinctively try to use orgasm to preserve our relationships and
counter the initial unpleasant effects of post-orgasmic hangovers.

However, due to the recurring aftereffects of excess dopamine, we are
pretty much doomed to eventual relationship deterioration. My sus-
picion is that this deterioration begins the very instant a hangover leads
us to imagine that our discomfort is due to our partner. Usually this
happens at a level we are not consciously aware of, but, even so, our
oxytocin drops off. Why? Because when we see someone as the cause
of our uneasiness, we no longer want to get closer. Our body chemistry swiftly aligns with our changed perception, producing a decrease
in bonding neurochemistry—and unfortunate neural reconfiguration.

Over time, this problem tends to catch up with every couple following biology's script unless they can overlook every uneasy feeling
(projection of uneasiness) they have about each other so the oxytocin
continues to flow. But unconditional forgiveness in the face of a steady
stream of subconscious, neurochemical hangovers is a tall order—
especially for a sober person. In my experience, it is easier to get around
the urge to separate with the two-step formula recommended in this
book:

- avoid overheating sexually (that is, maintain dopamine at moderate levels), and
- regularly exchange genuinely caring affection (to elevate oxytocin
  levels).

A Tough Lesson

Unfortunately, merely avoiding orgasm does not guarantee that dopamine levels remain within a comfortable range. Will and I learned this the hard way. Lulled into complacency by the easy harmony between us, we began making love whenever we felt like it instead of on a schedule, as recommended in Chapter 12.

Cracks appeared, but we did our best to ignore them. Without even noticing, we drifted away from the thoughtful exchanges of touch and more toward standard "let me feel you up" foreplay. Then our sleeping went out of sync. Will awakened earlier and earlier. If he got up and left for his office, it created an emotional rift between us, and if he stayed he was so restless that I felt obliged to try to comfort him. Both of us were usually exhausted by early evening.

My libido fell off to an alarming degree, but I did my best to remain sexually receptive, hoping that things would come back into balance when Will felt more nourished. Instead he grew hungrier. We sometimes made love when I was not really ready, in a misguided attempt to regain the closeness that was fading. To me it felt like I was nursing an increasingly demanding infant, and I was astonished at how draining it was—and resentful. He felt confused and frustrated. As he said, "I am only touching you as I always have, and if you now don't like it, you must not love me after all."

When I suggested that we back up and try the *Exchanges* again to shift our body chemistry away from the hunger cycle, it became obvious just how far off course we had blown. "If I tried to do what you are suggesting, I'd feel neutered," he cried. "You're trying to take away all my sexual pleasure!" Ugh. This did not sound like Will. After all, while doing the *Exchanges* and for months afterward, he had been amazed at how satisfied he felt, whether it was a lovemaking night or just a snuggle night. Why did his happiness and manhood now hinge on yielding to hungry impulses that were out of alignment with our original gains? What had we done wrong?

As it turned out, we had made a rather small mistake. When we stopped making love on a schedule, we unintentionally turned our controls back over to biology. Will, a typical, red-blooded male, is programmed to pursue all potential sexual opportunities. Without a schedule, it was his biological duty to rev up constantly . . . just in case. He was like a car engine that was semi-overheated all the time. His nervous system never got a chance to relax into the healing comfort of our initial time together, when we knew when we would and would not be having intercourse.

For such an innocent mistake it took surprisingly long to undo the damage. Not only had our future together come into doubt, but our mutual magnetism, which had once been utterly reliable, was not there to pull us back together. Ouch.

First we attempted to return to a schedule. That failed. No electricity was flowing, our hearts felt guarded, Will's touch was still hungry, I had a dream orgasm, which meant another two weeks of unbalanced energy. Sure enough, we got an unfair traffic ticket. My wallet was stolen. Crises at work drained our energy. The electrical power went out for days. Our lives seemed caught in a bizarre downward spiral on every front.

We realized that if what we had learned was correct, we would have to reorient our nervous systems completely . . . again . . . toward giving and away from craving, even though it meant another uncomfortable withdrawal period. We were badly frightened. As Will said, "I just don't think I can do it. I don't know how to touch you."

With heavy hearts we put our sleeping garb back on anyway and began the *Exchanges*. Could they work twice, especially given our state of mind? *Had they worked at all?* Every gain of the past year came into question. Maybe we had just been kidding ourselves. Maybe Will's addiction and depression had disappeared for other, unrelated reasons. Maybe there was no way to best biology. I felt doomed to become a "scaggy hag." Certainly the dark circles that had appeared under my eyes during the preceding weeks suggested there was no escape. Even my complexion had taken on a new pallor.

At first time stood still. Though we were both as caring and affectionate as possible, the *Exchanges* now felt dry as dust. Will made a concerted effort to avoid flipping on his dopamine hunger switch. Specifically, he touched my whole body as if one part were no more important than the other rather than focusing on his favorite bits.

Instead of concentrating on his own sensations, he tuned into my response to his touch. I made every effort to be affectionate and return his affection even when tired.

Within a couple of days things lightened up between us, but initially it felt like the camaraderie between condemned prisoners sharing a final meal. However, we were definitely sleeping better and better, and on the same schedule again. After about six or seven days Will felt a turning point, which he calls "the craving turning point." He felt noticeably calmer and less agitated. Our "I love you's" took on a new enthusiasm, and we laughed a lot. Both "intercourse" nights and "just snuggle" nights regained their former tenderness and contentment.

> When you love somebody, your eyelashes go up and down and little stars come out of you.
> —Karen, age 7

We felt optimistic again. Our careers took big jumps and we *looked* better. The last thing to recover was my libido. Clearly my subconscious had registered "feeling devoured" as a frightening experience, even though Will had never been aggressive or even openly demanding.

What did we learn from this ordeal? The pleasure/reward center of the brain is not designed for constant over-stimulation. In our experience, if we do not regulate ourselves, our bodies will self-regulate by driving us apart. That default solution is excruciating because uneasiness stops the flow of oxytocin. When your hearts slam shut it hurts.

Love & Fear

When oxytocin levels drop, you do not only feel unloving. You cut off oxytocin's other miraculous advantages. It seems that each month scientists discover another health benefit conferred by oxytocin. In order to understand how potent it really is, you will need to know something about a neurochemical whose damaging effects oxytocin counteracts. That is cortisol, the stress hormone.

As many observers of human nature have declared, we have only two basic emotions: love and fear. Just as joy, contentment, and benevolence are linked with open hearts or love, so grief, anger, and apathy signal underlying fear or closed hearts. Think of it this way: We have an enormous capacity for creative *thought,* but our bodies have only one basic *physical* choice: ease when we feel safe and loved, or stress when we feel endangered.

Oxytocin, as we have seen, is somewhat synonymous with *love.* My candidate for the fear hormone is *cortisol.* Cortisol levels rise significantly when we feel threatened. It is a vital neurochemical, with the power to keep us alive under severe conditions like starvation or critical injury, but at chronically high levels it is just plain harmful.

Cortisol is sometimes known as the death hormone because when it remains at high levels it ages us rapidly and lowers our immunity to disease. It literally turns muscle into fat and weakens bones. It is also associated with memory and concentration problems. Too much cortisol can lead to excitability, sleeplessness, and psychosis, and even damage the brain. As I found out, it can also reduce levels of estrogen and testosterone, leading to a drop in libido. And it no doubt had a lot to do with the dark circles and pallor that showed up in my face as our relationship seemed destined for the rocks.

> You have two choices in life: you can stay single and be miserable, or get married . . . and wish you were dead.
>
> —W.W. Renwick

Happily, oxytocin's healing effects on stress are so powerful that it may one day be known as the anti-stress hormone. It counteracts the changes brought on by cortisol. It allows us to think more clearly and cope with demands that we would otherwise find too much to face when under stress. It reduces the physical pain some people feel as stress levels increase. And it even diminishes the release of cortisol itself, which moderates our fight-or-flight response.[43] No wonder making love is such a good short-term antidote to stress.

Incidentally, much of lovemaking's benefit comes from touch itself. Caring touch, rather than eager fondling, raises oxytocin levels. It helps us heal faster and resist illness. For example, one month of regular massage for HIV-positive men significantly strengthened their embattled immune systems.[44] Compassionate touch has also been shown to reduce irritability and cravings by raising levels of a pleasure neurochemical called serotonin. It may even decrease the urge to ejaculate. (For example, Prozac users, who have artificially increased levels of serotonin, often experience delayed ejaculation without trying.) Touch also allows us to sleep more easily by reducing levels of adrenaline and cortisol.[45]

For women, enjoyment of intercourse is associated with longer life.[46] There is also less heart disease in women who are more satisfied with the quality of their sex lives.[47] And having sex twice per week appears to reduce the risk of death for men by half (compared with those who had sex once a month).[48] Ejaculation fans often cite this last study as proof that regular ejaculation prolongs men's lives, but the more than 900 study participants (age 45–59 at the beginning of the study) were virtually all making love with long-term female partners. Ejaculation and masturbation were not isolated as control factors; only sex with a partner was. So the study probably tells us more about the gains from regular intimate contact (and relative harmony) than the advantages of ejaculation itself.

Love Heals

When we learn to stay in love enough to stay close, we can do much to heal chronic stress-related misery. At present, 70 million Americans suffer from a condition resulting from excess cortisol known as Syndrome X.[49] The symptoms are excess weight, low energy, muddled thinking, high blood sugar, high cholesterol levels, and high blood pressure or even full-blown heart disease.

Everyone knows that stress increases the chance of heart disease. But it now appears that the primary mechanism behind this killer is *lowered oxytocin,* which allows cortisol to do its damage.[50] A study was done of almost ten thousand married men with chest pain (angina). Among those with high risk factors—elevated cholesterol, high blood pressure, age, diabetes, and irregular heartbeat—there was almost twice as much angina in the group of men who answered "No" to the question, "Does your wife show you her love?"[51]

Close to half of all Americans now die of heart disease, and apparently many of us are overlooking the best, most natural cure: loving relationships. As heart disease specialist Dean Ornish, M.D. explained in *Love & Survival,*[52] love and intimacy are such powerful determinants of health that if they came in drug form, doctors who failed to prescribe them would unquestionably be guilty of malpractice. In fact, he wrote that book to make the point that behaviors that connect us with others in a genuinely caring way have an even greater beneficial impact on our health than regular exercise, stopping smoking, or improved diet.

Oxytocin also protects against depression. Increased cortisol appears to be the major mechanism that causes depression. Some researchers suggest that Prozac and other antidepressants work by blocking cortisol's effects on the brain. It appears that oxytocin may work in a similar way, counteracting cortisol's negative effects on our minds, bodies, and relationships. Oxytocin may turn out to be our built-in, natural antidepressant.

> *Feelings of aliveness and vigor are the ultimate resources for the healing of trauma.* —*Peter Levine author of*
> Waking the Tiger: Healing Trauma

One of the most interesting bits of research about the benefits of union came out of a study measuring oxytocin levels in women in response to different stimuli. Participants' oxytocin levels were measured both while receiving a massage and while watching a sad movie. Some women in the study showed significantly greater increases in oxytocin in response to the massage, and they maintained higher levels of it in the face of sad emotions. When puzzled researchers investigated further, it turned out that these women were in couple relationships or had less anxiety in their relationships. Single women and those reporting interpersonal distress registered less benefit (i.e., less increase in oxytocin) from caring attention, and they were more depressed by sadness (i.e., more pronounced oxytocin decreases).[53]

It may be that when we grow despondent about intimacy, certain receptors on our nerve cells hibernate. And when we find a new sense of optimism about relationships, we activate these dormant receptors and produce oxytocin to promote bonding. Indeed, because the number of receptors on our nerve cells for neurochemicals associated with different emotions can change, we are not bound by our childhood patterns. We can physically reprogram ourselves for greater contentment. Such shifts may explain why people who have tried this recommended approach to sex discover an elation about getting closer that simply was not formerly in their repertoire. In short, some of us cannot accurately assess our potential for fulfilling intimacy until we take the first steps toward promoting different body chemistry by adopting a new behavior.

> *We've been practicing making love for several months this other way, and I haven't ejaculated once. I feel a lot better. I no longer have any guilt about sex, or worry about my performance. It makes me feel good to be so relaxed with her, without anxiety. During intercourse, we go for a little while and just relax together, and then repeat the cycle over and over. My health and my sense of well-being have changed for the better. I have quit drinking and cut way back on smoking. I have no back pain, heartburn, headaches, or elbow pain anymore. I'm sleeping better, and don't have frightening dream images like I had before.   —Matt*

Before leaving the healing properties of oxytocin, I should also touch on its power to reduce cravings. Rats addicted to heroin (which they could administer to themselves at will) were then treated with oxytocin. They showed a marked decrease in heroin use. Increased oxytocin levels also lessened various effects on cocaine-addicted rats, and even the symptoms of withdrawal from marijuana dependence.[54] So there is science behind my (and others') experience of lovers mastering addictions that previously ruled them.

Indeed, this hidden potential in harmonious couplehood may offer new encouragement for those facing some otherwise depressing statistics. Seventy percent of chronic problem drinkers are either divorced or separated. Single men are more than three times as likely as married men to die of cirrhosis of the liver.[55] Sexual relationships that heal can do much to improve these statistics.

Oxytocin's ability to relieve cravings probably also explains why we humans can get around our orgasm reflex without intense frustration or physical stress when we keep our oxytocin levels up with compassionate affection. But there is little progress without an open mind. One day as I started to catalog the rewards of avoiding ejaculation for a friend, he stopped me with "I've heard we can get prostate trouble from not ejaculating." When I did some research I learned that this widespread belief began when a study revealed that priests have a disproportionately high rate of prostate trouble.

I tracked the study down in a medical library. It turns out that prostate trouble is a function of congestion, which is stagnant blood. So frequent activity that moves the blood in the prostate region, not ejaculation itself, is the key to prostate health.[56] (Gay men, by the way, have a lower-than-average incidence of prostate trouble—and lots of prostate stimulation.) When I asked a medical doctor who has been studying Tantra for years about prostate trouble and ejaculation, he said, "I don't know of any further research on this, but I have a strong opinion that the big consideration is whether there is a sense of control/frustration/holding back involved. If one is moving energy well, then congestion does not happen."

With the approach I am recommending, lovers tend to make love for longer periods of time and more often, without becoming uncomfortably over-aroused. Also, erections come and go, which gently pumps blood through the entire prostate region. Most importantly, both partners produce an enhanced body chemistry that helps ward off all disease.

A Fountain of Youth, the Ultimate Diet, and an All-Purpose Healing Tonic

The advantages of harmonious union are considerable, thanks largely to oxytocin. Decades of research have firmly established that a stable, happy marriage is the best defense against illness and premature death.[57] In a seven-year study of 800 young adults, depression and alcohol abuse declined more significantly for those who married during that time.[58] Co-habitors, too, enjoy significantly lower levels of psychological distress than individuals with no partner or those with a partner living outside the household.[59]

To be sure, it is not the marriage certificate or shared address that protects you. Indeed, as we will see in Chapter 6, both marital disharmony and divorce correlate with poorer health. So the benefits of union hinge on couples maintaining a degree of harmony.[60] Science has begun to measure the gifts of togetherness. For example, studies done over two decades involving more than thirty-seven thousand people show that social isolation—the sense that you have nobody with whom you can share your private feelings or have close contact—doubles the chances of sickness or death.[61]

Love is what makes you smile when you're tired. —Terri, age 4

Researchers are also beginning to measure the gains from intimacy's less tangible aspects, such as the benefits that come from caring about another. For example, in primate species where the male is the primary caregiver, males live longer than females and vice versa.[62] And a soon-to-be released University of Michigan study of hundreds of older couples found that engaging in altruistic behavior increases longevity. Over a five-year period, the givers were 40 to 60 percent less likely to die. Spouses who were able to make their spouse feel loved and cared for also lived longer than those who gave no emotional support.[63] Those who help others also report a helper's high, a euphoria so powerful that it can ease the symptoms of stress-related disorders such as headaches, voice loss, and pain accompanying lupus and multiple sclerosis. The feel-good sensation is most intense when actually touching or listening to someone.[64] It is easy to see how this joy from giving can bring about deeper bonding and ecstatic feelings between lovers.

Three weeks after we began the Exchanges, *my libido started to return. In the months since, my health has steadily improved, my energy level has risen, and my sexual desire has continued to increase. I'm happy. My friends comment that I'm glowing and look 10–15 years younger.*   —Ellen

---

The returns on openheartedness are so unmistakable that scientists have now begun looking for practical ways to boost oxytocin and lower cortisol. For example, the Institute of HeartMath has demonstrated that consciously choosing emotions of caring, compassion, and appreciation has measurable health advantages.[65] After a month, people who were taught to substitute these positive feelings for feelings of anger and frustration showed significant beneficial changes in key hormone levels. So it is not unreasonable to conclude that learning to make giving the focus in our intimate relationships is excellent health insurance.

Social ties are the cheapest medicine we have.
  —*Shelley Taylor, author of* The Tending Instinct

Did you know that the ancient Chinese Taoists prescribed hours of non-orgasmic sex in various positions as cures for a host of diseases? Imagine doctors' prescriptions reading, "Patient must stay home and make love all day for serious health reasons." Even better than a hand-icapped parking sticker!

The Taoists also claimed that correct mutual cultivation of sexual energy could lead to immortality. So HeartMath's findings that caring and appreciation raised levels of the anti-aging hormone, DHEA, are especially intriguing. DHEA is closely linked to our sexual vitality because it is the precursor to the sex hormones estrogen and testosterone. In short, if you want to feel young and sexy, shift your focus to nurturing your partner with an open heart and ignore biology's fertilization behavior commands.

Synchronizing Hearts

Openheartedness is not merely an aid in bonding deeply and a means of staying youthful, fit, and more resistant to disease. The heart has another hidden talent. It generates the strongest electromagnetic field that the body produces. In fact, it can be measured up to ten feet beyond the body. HeartMath has also shown that this field becomes measurably more coherent as we shift to sincerely loving or caring states. Coherence is an indication of inner balance. It means that our body systems are working especially well together. It correlates with increased immunity, clearer thinking, and the capacity to handle stress more easily with greater flexibility. Our bodies clearly like equilibrium.

Best of all, a coherent electromagnetic heart field may be the key to truly remarkable states of union. When we touch someone while in a loving, coherent state, our heartbeat can even register in his/her brain waves.[66] This potential for synchronizing electromagnetic fields when in a loving state may account for the Taoist Valley Orgasm experience in which lovers sense a profound merging that leaves them tingling with well-being for days or weeks.

Suddenly we both seemed to be floating in an unbounded space filled with warmth and light. The boundaries between our bodies dissolved and, along with them, the distinctions between man and woman. We were one. The experience became timeless, and we seemed to remain like this forever. There was no need to have an orgasm. There was no need even to "make love." There was nothing to do, nothing to achieve. We were in ecstasy.
—*Margo Anand, author of* The Art of Sexual Ecstasy

HeartMath has yet to do any research on comparing different approaches to sex. However, Rollin McCraty, Director of Research at HeartMath Institute, told me that he once measured the heart rate coherence over a 24-hour period for a number of couples attending a Tantra workshop. He found that there was an unexpectedly high incidence of synchronization between some partners—especially while they were sleeping. As you will see, the *Exchanges* in Chapter 12 begin with sleeping together. Experience has shown that this gentle contact has very beneficial effects, some of which may come from this subconscious synchronization between open hearts.

Partner Pampering

Try for a moment to feel *love* and *hate* at the same time. You cannot. In fact, there is no middle ground between an open heart and a closed one, and very different body chemistry accompanies each. This means that the cure for unhealthy defensiveness is not neutrality, or even negotiated fairness. It is active caring or giving. You have to move your attention outward to reap the rewards of an open heart.

It is thus impossible to mix the reward-seeking of conventional sex with the approach advocated in this book and see lasting gains. If we do not consistently tap the body chemistry gifts of openhearted caring in our relationships, we are stuck in neutral. Then we naturally tend to seek even harder for fulfillment through greater passion. Ultimately biology succeeds in pushing us back into conventional orgasm and a downward spiral.

Conscious giving is the best defense against impulsive behavior. You may have forgotten how wonderful it feels to care for your partner thoughtfully because conventional sex so swiftly makes relationships mutually draining. This feeling of being drained, of course, is what makes us defensive and unenthusiastic about giving. This biological selfishness has haunted us for a long time and has profound spiritual implications, which I will address in Chapter 8.

The good news is that when you make love without this drain, giving soon becomes a habit. Why? It feels good, thanks to oxytocin. Your partner's joy is yours as well. Mutual caring creates a profound feeling of comfort and a sense of abundance. Old fears of intimacy simply cannot withstand this deep sense of mutual security, so they fade away.

When someone loves you, the way they say your name is different. You know that your name is safe in their mouth.

—Billy, age 4

Focusing your attention on making your partner feel loved is also a reliable aphrodisiac. While traditional foreplay is often about purchasing sex and eventually leaves someone unhappy with the bargain, a loving head rub or foot rub, without expectations, is truly a gift. Genuine gifts call forth a spontaneous receptivity and desire for merging from your partner—and that is always a turn-on.

A friend in England who experimented with a variation of the *Exchanges* found that soon she enthusiastically initiated sex with her husband, which he relished. For years she had grimly endured intercourse, which she had found painful, just to hold her marriage together. "And," she confided in her colorful Cockney accent, "'E *loved* 'es foot massage. In twenty-foive years of marriage oi'd never even *seen* 'es feet!"

When you take the biological goal of conventional orgasm out of sex, it frees you to approach each other more selflessly. It is heartening to know that your partner is looking out for you and has the boundless energy of a teen to do it. You can also explore new heights of intimacy when you can both surrender in safety. Effortlessness pervades relationships built on this foundation. There is no performance anxiety and, obviously, no pressure on either lover to deliver an orgasm to please a partner.

The healing that follows this simple change of heart from "what can I get?" to "what can I give?" will genuinely astound you. Setbacks that would be cause for outrage if you were thinking of your partnership as a deal are only cause for compassion and assistance if your motivation is to comfort and heal. Needless to say, we recover from bad habits far more rapidly without recrimination or guilt in the mix.

It is impossible to appreciate fully the peace of mind and increase in well-being that accompanies this approach until you try it for an extended period. At first, though, you will need a very slow, conservative approach to sexual intimacy. Remember when you learned to ride a bicycle? At first it was nerve-wracking, but you soon came to love the feeling of perfect balance, freedom, and control. When this new approach becomes automatic, sexual arousal will no longer demand frantic fertilization efforts. Instead it will feel like an invitation to enter into a steady state of delicious, satisfying lovemaking that has a timeless, fulfilling, eternal quality to it. Best of all, you can produce the body chemistry that accompanies it indefinitely. It is far better for you than the explosive, imbalanced body chemistry that biology orchestrates to meet its goals.

> *At first when I realized my lover was more generous than I was, I felt like the right answer was for her to give less. I see now that that would have slowly strangled the relationship by setting up a constant negotiation about who was doing more. I'm glad I discovered true giving. I feel stronger, more confident, and more ... connected to the universal flow. The more I give, the more comes my way—from everywhere.*   —*Bruce*

Summary

- ❧ Oxytocin is the neurochemical associated with love. It is behind emotional bonding and the desire to nurture.
- ❧ Cortisol is the neurochemical associated with fear. In excess it is associated with the undesirable health effects of stress.
- ❧ It is easier to keep dopamine, the craving neurochemical, at moderate levels when you make love on a schedule with pre-determined breaks in it.
- ❧ Oxytocin counteracts the effects of cortisol and also lessens cravings.
- ❧ Making love with the intention to heal each other keeps oxytocin levels high and improves both givers' health.

The Marshmallow Challenge

Some years back, a group of four-year-olds was offered the following proposition: "If you wait till I run an errand, you can have two marshmallows. If you can't wait, you can have only one—but you can have it right now." The choices these children made revealed their trajectory through life. According to Daniel Goleman in *Emotional Intelligence*,[67] the capacity to resist impulse is the root of all emotional self-control. The primitive brain acts on reflex, while the higher brain sees consequences.

The four-year-olds who were able to wait resisted temptation by covering their eyes so they would not have to stare at the bait, rested their heads in their arms, talked, sang, played games with their hands and feet, or even tried to sleep. The more impulsive ones grabbed the marshmallow, almost always within seconds of the experimenter's departure on his twenty-minute "errand."

Twelve to fourteen years later, the difference between the two groups was dramatic. Those who had resisted temptation were now more personally effective, self-assertive, and better able to cope with life's frustrations. They were less likely to go to pieces under stress, or to become rattled and disorganized when pressured; they pursued challenges even in the face of difficulties; they were self-reliant, confident, trustworthy, dependable, and far superior as students—regardless of IQ.

The grabbers, however, were more likely to shy from social contact; to be stubborn and indecisive; to be easily upset by frustration; to think of themselves as "bad" or unworthy; to become immobilized by stress; to be mistrustful and resentful about not getting enough; to be prone to jealousy and envy; to overreact with a sharp temper, provoking arguments and fights. And they were *still* unable to put off immediate gratification in pursuit of other goals. Because of their over-active pleasure/reward centers, I would be willing to bet that they also masturbated more frequently . . . bless their hearts.

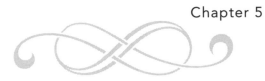

Chapter 5

Outwitting Biology

THIS CHAPTER ADDRESSES SOME OF THE WAYS OUR biological programming has brainwashed us and impaired our capacity for intimacy. Awareness and a new approach to sex can help us steer around the iceberg of biologically driven sex. The visible part of the iceberg is temptation, but the more treacherous portion lies beneath the surface in the form of subconscious, misplaced danger signals.

When it comes to sex, we have all learned to grab for the one marshmallow. Of course, some of us have mastered the use of birth control, and the world-class lovers among us have learned to orchestrate simultaneous orgasms. Yet even our efforts at self-control have revolved around the ultimate objective of grabbing the dopamine blast in the form of conventional orgasm. This is why we seldom tap the most precious gifts of sexual self-discipline: healing and harmony. Our primitive brain can impel sexual behavior and record painful experiences, but it does not *consciously choose*. Fortunately it is possible to recondition the brain to develop a new set of reflexes.

Still, let's face it. Tempting as a marshmallow may be to a four-year-old, it holds little allure compared with an orgasm for many. So if you decide to learn to make love this other way, and conventional sex is a favorite pastime, you face a challenge. You must resolutely tune out the insistent signals of your limbic system, which has had the upper hand for a long time when it comes to sexual response.

This can be done, and as you will see if you try the *Exchanges,* I recommend many of the same techniques the savvy four-year-olds employed. Instead of covering your eyes, you simply keep some clothing on for a while. You, too, distract yourself with carefully chosen activities so you have something to do with your sexual desire other than follow your impulses to their natural conclusion. And you nourish and balance each other by exchanging affection and sleeping together. When intercourse enters the picture, you steer around temptation by avoiding vigorous movement. Each *Exchange* also offers a pep talk, because no matter how much you are drawn to the ideas in this book, your primitive brain guarantees a very short memory about why you are passing up that marshmallow.

If you were a one-marshmallow kid, beware of your inner rebel. You may be used to giving in to energy-draining impulses that do not truly satisfy, such as eating chocolate or sugary foods, drinking alcohol, masturbating, smoking, hot foreplay, or getting lost in television or pulp novels. It is easy to mistake such gut-level cravings for your true will. Voluntarily adopting a daily recipe like the *Exchanges* is a way of countering the hold of any self-destructive appetites. The rewards of self-control are accessible, but they depend upon willingness.

Seek Not the Solution Where the Answer Is Barred

When I was first learning about the benefits of avoiding orgasm, I happened to see a television program about sexual issues called "Strictly Personal." The topic was, "Men Who Fake Orgasm." An attractive guy in his thirties explained that he really enjoys making love but does not always want to come. His girlfriend, however, convinced him that she feels unattractive and unloved if he does not orgasm. So he uses a condom, fakes the orgasm, and discards the (missing) evidence. A guest sexologist then explained why his instinctively correct, healing behavior was "a problem" according to her training.

The day after I saw the show I happened to be on a long flight seated next to two friendly, macho Italian-American construction workers in their thirties who were close friends. When I told them about the show, one of them burst out laughing, "Ha, ha, ha! Men who fake orgasm! That's the funniest thing I ever heard."

His best buddy turned to him and said, "I've done that."

Sexologists have been trained to diagnose any deviation from biologically driven sexual behavior as a problem. Therefore men who prefer to avoid ejaculation and women who do not snap at every opportunity to climax are suspect. The experts may be basing their advice on complaints they hear from clients who come to them because of problems with conventional sex. Apparently they hear a lot of complaints, too: forty-three percent of women and thirty-one percent of men experience sexual difficulties.[68]

I think it will turn out that a misplaced focus on orgasm is the culprit behind most of these difficulties, and that these troubles are loud signals that we have the wrong goals in bed. After all, at least ninety-nine percent of sexual encounters take place without the intention to fertilize an ovum. When we insist on engaging in sexual behavior that is fertilization-driven (and disquieting), it is like continuing to eat high-calorie desserts because one percent of the population wants to gain weight.

> Because over the past few years, more money has been spent on breast implants and Viagra than is spent on Alzheimer's Disease research, it is believed that by the year 2030 there will be a large number of people wandering around with huge breasts and erections ... who can't remember what to do with them.
>
> —Andy Rooney

In my experience, men can recover from premature ejaculation or increase their libido, and women can grow more sexually responsive and avoid urinary tract infection with a different approach to sex. I believe that statistical studies will bear out such experiences on a large scale as soon as we are willing to conduct the necessary research.

Blind indulgence is not the only definition of "normal" when it comes to sex. True, someone who does not completely open physically and emotionally to his or her partner has blocked energy. But as that block is often at the heart, enticements for heating up our genitals temporarily mask, rather than solve, any underlying uneasiness.

In my experience, a relationship based strictly on mutual caring and safety is a rapid, effective way to open hearts. Later portions of this book abound with practical suggestions for how to move in this direction. As your hearts open, you both effortlessly attune to each other at very subtle levels. This makes your lovemaking as elegant as a ballet but with the lighthearted flirtatiousness of a spring picnic *à deux* and the emotional depth of a great novel. I suspect that this heightened sensitivity is the very key to satisfying ecstasy without energy hangovers.

> Statistics, as you know, is the most exact of false sciences.
> —Jean Cau

You will always have the option of using your newfound openness for conventional sex if you want to be *normal,* but that choice will also carry you back into a *natural* addictive cycle followed by the *usual* separation. So do not be afraid to chart new territory. The statistics will catch up with those of us who master this new approach.

How Do I Know if Biology is Pulling My Strings ... Again?

Good intentions are not enough to divert you from the primitive pull toward fertilization-based sex. And it can be difficult to know when you are on the right track. The chart on the opposite page contains some helpful comparisons.

Happily, men who make up their minds to pass up orgasm achieve their goal fairly easily with a loving partner. Even if they have been ejaculating frequently, within a few days the neurochemical command to fertilize quiets down. Perhaps it is because the hormone vasopressin reaches ideal levels. Vasopressin appears to make males protective of their mates and aids memory (helping them remember why they want to wait for that second marshmallow?). That is the good news.

The bad news is that self-control during intercourse does not come as effortlessly to women. They, after all, are on the receiving end of things. Also, their open vulnerability actually assists their mates in controlling themselves because it furnishes them with what they most need

CONVENTIONAL SEX	HEALING SEX
Impulsive, spur-of-the moment lovemaking	Gradual, conscious preparation prior to making love
Rapid movement	Emphasis on stillness
Tension	Relaxation
Urgent need for release	No need for release
Rapid conclusion	Prolonged union of cycles, erection comes and goes
Urgency to achieve a goal	Playfulness, ease in staying in the present, never hurried
Feelings of "I want," "I must have," or hunger	Can make love with enthusiasm, or defer without disappointment
Sex is just sex	Sex is a delicious experience of companionship and comfort
Sense that partner is trying to control you, "move too fast," or will abandon you	Sense of gratitude for time spent together. You feel very fortunate.
Avoidance of closer union—due to projection of sense of deprivation or uneasiness onto partner	Desire for closer union—due to projection of increasing sense of well-being onto partner

from the encounter. As relationship expert John Gray put it, "A man is empowered and nurtured most when he feels appreciated, accepted and trusted. . . . When a woman is longing to have sex with a man, she is most open and trusting. In a very dramatic way, she is willing to surrender her defenses. . . ."[69] In keeping with women's open role, they apparently gush with cuddly oxytocin, and little vasopressin.

Most women do not start out as orgasm-prone during intercourse as men. Shere Hite (*The Hite Report,* 1976) found that only thirty percent of the women who responded to her questionnaire reached orgasm regularly from intercourse alone. However, using sex to heal seems to open everyone at deeper levels, so women grow increasingly sensitive and responsive. Since women are ideally in a more receptive role energetically, this can spell trouble. For example, I have found that if my partner slides toward physical gratification I slide right with him, and soon climax, with little or no warning. If his intentions are purely to nurture me safely, however, my control improves. In other words, his intentions are more critical to my maintaining balance than his actions, and I am sure my intentions also affect his degree of control.

Perilous Passion

Control is not the biggest challenge you face when you move away from your biological blueprint toward a healing relationship. The biggest challenge is the millennia of distrust between the sexes caused by conventional sex. Deep in our collective unconscious, passion has a bad rap. That is, tasty as that passion marshmallow is, it is also associated with subsequent chaos, emotional distress, and even spiritual demotion according to such diverse authorities as Adam & Eve and the Tibetan Buddhists.

At first I was skeptical about this passion/fear connection, but clues abound. Here is one that a friend sent me from an English newspaper:

> The Hulis, aborigines of New Guinea, also known as "Wig Men," have a traditional distrust of women, believing that females take their powers from them. As a result they live apart from their bare-breasted wives and cook their own food. Sex is reduced to a brief encounter.

Crude superstition? Perhaps. However, one Western, lusty bachelor who assured me he was typical summarized his sexual routine as "Get on, get off, get home." Incidentally, he has also learned to cook his own food since his divorce. Apparently some Wig Men are not wearing wigs. Maybe the Hulis are not as peculiar as we suppose.

Although we consciously associate passion with pleasure, another portion of our primitive brain views passion as suicidal. I believe that this subconscious association accounts for the potency of the emotional rift between the sexes. Sex is the hub of the birth/death wheel.

It brings us onto the planet, and it is indirectly responsible for taking us off, too. It succeeds by gradually causing us to separate from each other, thus cutting ourselves off from our best source of rejuvenation (and decreasing production of oxytocin and anti-aging hormone DHEA). If our relationship is stressful on top of it, we hasten our physical decline with lethal levels of cortisol.

> Sexual pleasure is not, in principle, wrong. However, . . . conventional pleasure is associated with the loss of life-energy. In your casual adaptation, pleasure and death, sex and death, eroticism and death, have always been felt to be the same event. You must, in your right emotional and sexual adaptation, discover the pleasure that is inherent in life.[70]

The French refer to ejaculation as *la petite mort,* or the little death. If you ejaculate into your partner, the link between sex and this little death is projected onto her. Men who get the urge to bolt after sex are not jerks; they just cannot face being chained to someone who is starting to look a little like a skull and crossbones until death do us part. Of course, running away merely cuts them off from the potential advantages of union and guarantees them the same problem when their next "need for intimacy" (as relationship guru John Gray so delicately puts it) drives them into another encounter.

Not all of them run. Some, in obedience to this reflex of decline, begin to ensure their deterioration through illness, addiction, or impotence. Like men, women often unconsciously create distance in relationships to ward off the stress of conventional sex. It does not matter how they do it: moodiness, hurt feelings, accusations, weight gain, unreasonable demands, irrational fears, illness, needing space, or growing in different directions. The bottom line is separation.

> Food has replaced sex in my life. Now I can't even get into my own pants.

The pursuit of genital orgasm seduces men and women into running on short-life batteries instead of staying plugged into an inexhaustible source of strength and inspiration. And we do not even realize there is an alternative until we learn to sustain a heart link with a partner. That grows increasingly unlikely as we continue to hit this raw nerve of fear in our subconscious.

Consider *Romeo and Juliet* or *The English Patient*. Even our art reflects a connection between passion and disaster. It is no wonder we often see the world as a place of decay and despair. Since I have become more observant of this connection between passion and decline, I have begun to notice how often a philosophy of gloom sets in during the weeks following a passion bout.

The Key to Mortality

A hangover from too much passion (or masturbation) may even take the form of severe depression or a desire to commit suicide, which we never consciously associate with sex. Not only do I experience uncharacteristic discouragement, men who normally exude energy, optimism, and physical fitness will cynically explain to me that they do not want to live forever anyway to justify returning to a self-destructive habit or the abandonment of plans for personal growth they had eagerly anticipated. This despair is normal for many, but avoidable if we opt for an alternative approach to intimacy.

The reverse is also true. When making love without succumbing to biology's plan, both men and I who try the ideas astonish ourselves with our productivity, insight, cheerfulness, sexiness, youthfulness, and confidence. So I am convinced that we can evade biology's trap. For now, however, when genital orgasm creates feelings of dying a little, our body chemistry obediently responds by killing us a little. And this constant reminder of death seduces most of us into thoughts like: "We're all going to die anyway, so why not have a little pleasure first?" Indeed, perhaps you are beginning to see how conventional orgasm can bring about all the dire consequences that Eastern yogis warn of: weakness, lack of courage, and premature death. It is because of the uneasy body chemistry that eventually follows the sensation of let-down or emptiness after the high of orgasm.

I remember having been rather frightened as a boy when I first learned of examples in the animal world where the males die after having given away their sperm to procreate, e.g. the drones after the "marriage flight" with the queen. What was so dangerous about marriage and sex?   —*Stephen*

Some men report a different experience. Rather than a let-down, they may feel a frenzied euphoria after orgasm. The pursuit of orgasm may, in fact, cause them to seek dangerous thrills. The rush of PEA (stimulating stress hormone) that is so often present in initial sexual encounters is also released in large quantities during the free fall of a parachute jump. Some researchers surmise that this rush may be addictive, perhaps due to the increase in dopamine that accompanies it.

I once read that the group who will most likely die accidental and violent deaths is men in their twenties. It is worthy of note that a sort of death wish is most powerful when their sex drive is highest and their inclination to stay with a partner long enough to awaken more beneficial ecstatic body chemistry lowest. Higher testosterone levels during these years make both restlessness and the pursuit of sexual (fertilization) opportunities more probable. Incidentally, according to a recent study by the University of Arizona, both sexes in the age group 25–39 feel the most stress from interpersonal tension and disagreements with lovers, co-workers, and friends.[71] Could it be because this group is most sexually active?

At any rate, the real tragedy of the association between passion and feeling threatened is that it does not get better over time. Each sexual encounter reawakens it. Or the couple unconsciously avoids sex altogether to keep from triggering it, causing an unhealthy stagnation. If they stay together, their relationship becomes an empty shell. I know of one couple who now see each other every three weeks or so. They call it graceful distance. But all too often this subconscious uneasiness leaves us with a protective urge to grab the sex and avoid the intimacy.

So there you have the Key to Mortality. We each arrive here as a male or a female. And when we use or disuse sex in a way that does not promote harmony, the separation causes us to age more rapidly than we need to or go out with a flash. Rest assured that if you are currently scared to death of intimacy, you are not alone. But take heart in knowing that you are surrounded by millions of opportunities to reverse this unhealthy trajectory and escape biology's plans for you.

My Spouse Changed *Completely* After We Got Married

You do not have to allow biology to create inner conflict, but you will have to win your struggle from within with the help of a caring partner. Reconfigure your neural reflexes relating to sexual intimacy by producing lots of cuddle hormones while avoiding excess dopamine entirely. That way you literally choose rejuvenation instead of activating all the fear-based stuff that your subconscious associates with sex when passion is your objective.

You may still see some of your old defensive patterns for a while, but you will see them with greater detachment than you ever thought possible. They will not have the same ominous subconscious charge behind them. And when you look back a few months down the road, you will find you have discarded them with remarkable ease.

Of course, the pro-fertilization, passion track remains in your brain, subject to reactivation. So if you stray back into passion, you will swiftly set off your old alarms, even if no one has an actual orgasm. Your partner may suddenly bear a striking resemblance to all your partners from failed past relationships (rolled into one decidedly scary-looking creature). And your familiar, knee-jerk defenses to intimacy will arise.

This occurs, you may recall, because a part of your primitive brain, the amygdala, has very efficiently recorded your past, unhappy emotional fallout from the pursuit of passion. It cannot stop the impulsive sexual behavior mandated by other portions of the primitive brain (though you can when you learn to resist that marshmallow), but it can do an excellent job of defending you from ongoing intimacy.

Remember that your amygdala may well regard commitment to your partner as the gravest threat related to intimacy. When you commit, you tie yourself to a recurring sense of deprivation, at least while biology still pilots you. Your amygdala, therefore, increases its alarm volume, creating stress and dis-

Before you're married he'll help you over a straw. After you're married you can find your own way over a haystack.
—Country proverb

torting your perception of each other. I believe this perfectly under-standable defense mechanism accounts for the familiar cry, "My spouse changed completely after we got married."

The Intimacy Sabotaging Device

In more than ten years of watching others and myself, I never fail to be amazed at the efficacy of an amygdala pro-grammed to fear intimacy. Its voice is loud and its advice is lousy. It is utterly single-minded, and its goal, once triggered by hot sex, is to create separation between lovers, however it can. As I mentioned earlier, it sends its red-alert messages out in the form of stress chemicals before we can even analyze its suggestions with our more evolved brain lobes. The effects linger, too. I notice the effects of a passion hangover for at least two weeks after a conventional orgasm. And it usually gets worse just before it gets significantly better.

In effect, we possess an Intimacy Sabotaging Device, the purpose of which is to guard us against deepening intimacy after we have engaged in passion. As we age it becomes increasingly mechanical and reliable. The only way I have found to escape its control is not to pull its trigger. I make up my mind that my lover is regrettably not a marsh-mallow. He is in my arms to be healed. Period. Humanity has seldom used sex to heal, so our subconscious has no flashing danger signals related to such a foreign activity. And, humor aside, the rewards from giving are greater than those from receiving.

The Amygdala at Work
Yesterday Heidi, the woman I met on a bike tour, called me. We talked for two hours. When she learned that my birthday is com-ing up she wanted to celebrate it with me. I felt "attacked by surprise" and "breathless." I wanted to hammer her back, away from me. I told her I would prefer to make a bike tour ALONE on my birthday. It is so subconscious. I did not realize at first what I had done again.

There is always the feeling that if I engage too much in ANY relationship I will be imprisoned somehow and won't be able to be my own master, etc. How can I put my hammer aside and learn to interact with people better? There is so much I want to give, but it always ends with me standing alone with empty hands ... without having given anything.   —Gerhard

To Heal, Give

It is very difficult to fight a subconscious block and win. It is far easier to deflate it by channeling your energy in a new direction (while also strengthening your inner equilibrium). Try giving. As we saw in the last chapter, openhearted, caring emotions increase oxytocin levels, which protect our health and make us feel safe instead of threatened. To gain the upper hand over biology we must see our relationships differently.

At present we think of relationships as arm's-length deals. Even an ideal mate list is a catalog of the returns we are looking for on our potential investment. Historically this mentality has been viewed as great wisdom. In fact, until this century, most marriages were arranged for the participants so they would not let romantic nonsense get in the way of more sensible considerations. If there were no hidden potential between open hearts, such logic would make perfect sense. However, there is logic behind unselfish giving in relationships. In fact, here is an even more reliable returns principle than making deals: what you give out will return to you.

Solid relationships are built on what you each give. Indeed, you cannot build a solid relationship on what you each want. I am not talking about mutual sacrifice or about mutual selfishness, euphemistically known as negotiation. I am talking about a completely different flow of energy between partners than we see in conventional relationships.

The best way to feel satisfied, safe, and loved is to offer these gifts to your partner unconditionally. See your interests as equally important to both of you. Think of yourselves as two hands of one shared entity. There need not be a defensive sense of separation even though you are in two bodies. This shift toward a unified perception may take a while, but it requires surprisingly little effort when you consistently use this alternative approach to lovemaking. Less struggle also means more durable relationships.

Mutual altruism is a very high standard of conduct. I suspect it is impossible to maintain with conventional sex in the picture. While biology drives me, I just do not have the energy to put another first for long. The neurochemical storms and hangovers from fertilization-driven behavior create an artificial sense of deprivation. I can only think about what I personally need. It seems like someone is making unreasonable demands or like I am the victim of someone else's impossible behavior. I begin to perceive our interests as separate, and it feels like we are locked in a power struggle. The relationship takes on a suffocating quality.

> The best way to a man's heart is to saw his breastplate open.

This shutdown at the heart level is the highest price we pay for allowing our primitive brains to run our love lives. Not only does it affect our health adversely, but also we often become selfish or hopelessly judgmental. We have a powerful urge to separate to protect ourselves.

Meanwhile, if you have an ideal mate checklist, lose it . . . or become it. Giving without ulterior motive not only shifts your vision, but improves your health. No one will look more ideal to you than someone whose well-being you genuinely treasure.

Natural Euphoria

You may be thinking that sexual frustration itself is stressful. It is. But do not assume that you will be sexually frustrated simply because you and your partner avoid orgasm. If the solution I propose does not heal frustration it is no solution at all. Try the *Exchanges* completely, however, before you evaluate their effectiveness. A deep sense of well-being arises when you stop goal-oriented sexual behavior and just nurture each other for an extended period. As Taoists discovered thousands of years ago, your body can produce a most satisfying sex life without conventional orgasm.

Recent research suggests that true satisfaction is a function of what author William Bloom calls the endorphin effect.[72] Endorphins (endogenous morphine), the body's natural opiates, create physical pleasure and can ease pain more effectively than chemical morphine. They boost the immune system, speed the healing of damaged tissue, and create physical feelings of well-being. They are also behind the euphoria in which people experience a deep spiritual connection with others, all nature, and the universe. Many of the scientifically documented benefits of meditation are apparently due to increased endorphins. Lovemaking, too, can release them, at least until biology causes us to close our hearts in defensiveness.

> A man says (proudly) to his friend, "My wife's an angel!" "You're lucky," says his friend, "mine's still alive."

When we move away from biology's fertilization agenda we can relax into a state that feels like a whole different realm. In fact, scientists hypothesize that oxytocin, the cuddle hormone we examined in the previous chapter, may encourage bonding because of its calming effect on lovers. Perhaps there is some link between oxytocin and the production of endorphins. All I know is that when I am in this peaceful condition, I have the sense that my needs are effortlessly being met. I do not have to struggle and yet I have plenty of energy for things I feel called upon to undertake. This state of mind is deeply satisfying—and the key to escaping biology's clutches for good.

It also gives us lovers the strength to drop defensive patterns we chose in the past, such as shutting down emotionally, dissolving into tears, blaming or judging, substance addictions, or self-absorption. We realize that these old behaviors were not our true identity; they were just the way we closed our hearts when feeling deprived. It becomes apparent that the cure for many ills has always been to open our hearts and move toward (safer) union.

Lack

While we follow biology's plan, and our ecstasy is linked only to chemical blasts that we engineer, then whenever we are not high we feel like something is missing. Worse yet, our loving feelings are tangled up with artificial, forced jolts of pleasure. So when the inevitable hangovers arrive and we suddenly feel inexplicably awful, we imagine we have fallen out of love. It seems like our lover does not care enough to make us feel good again. Anger and resentment can lead to feelings of hate and powerful cravings for emotion-numbing substances or activities. This is the recurring seesaw of conventional relationships.

Many of us are familiar with spiritual authorities (Eckhart Tolle, for example) who warn against the addictive nature of romantic involvement. When you seek outside yourself, they assure us, you are bound to create a painful experience. Such authorities are not envisioning a relationship based on mutual giving. They are envisioning mutual *seeking* (that is, attempts to *get*). Certainly intimate relationships have long revolved around conventional sexual activity and the selfishness it fuels.

It is easy to see that we will always come up short if we use each other, albeit unintentionally, to create an artificial sense of lack, and then use each other to attempt to fill that very emptiness. Many spiritual traditions have assumed that the only way off the treadmill of empty obsessions and perpetual dissatisfaction is celibacy. Now, however, some spiritual advisors encourage us to stay in our mutually draining relationships until we exceed our pain threshold, separate, and devote ourselves to seeking within instead.

I no longer believe that the source of our distress is intimate contact. The problem is approaching each other while feeling greedy or needy. Our hunger can be due to isolation, overheating, or frequent orgasm—although a certain longing for wholeness accompanies the simple fact of being one gender or the other. Each of us is, after all, somewhat polarized, like half a magnet.

Once we resolve the situation so that there is no longer a sense of lack associated with union, we are free to discover the synergy and spiritual potential

One day I got two emails entitled, "FINALLY! A CHAIN LETTER WORTH READING." A man's version came from a guy and a woman's version from a girlfriend. The instructions said to add your name to the bottom of a list and send the chain letter to all your friends. Then you were to pack your lover in a box and send him/her to the name at the top of the list. Within weeks you would receive thousands of potential lovers to sort through and surely a few would be worth keeping . . . assuming everyone remembered to put air holes in the boxes. Brilliant, eh? Problem is, with our current sexual habits, we would soon be packing each other again. Improving our odds does not solve this syndrome. We have to heal the subconscious association of intimacy with uneasiness.

Don't think you can change
a man ... unless he's in
diapers.

that lies in mutual strengthening. We are still solving the problem from *within,* but not in isolation. We each solve it by balancing and stabilizing our magnetic attraction when we nurture another in a shared experience.

The suggestion that all spiritual work can be done far more efficiently solo (except for painful lessons with each other) is misguided. The return to full spiritual awareness is an experience of the truth that we are all one. A blissful merging with another ego at an energetic level is a very efficient shortcut to a state of mind in which we welcome our oneness with others.

Think Big

Changing the way we make love may have major implications. Just about everyone makes love or is influenced by people affected by lovemaking's familiar fallout. I now believe that the sociological and economic explanations for human behavior that I have studied are incomplete. They are addressing symptoms of a more fundamental cause: our chronic sense of deprivation. By self-inducing this condition we all contribute to humanity's greed, manipulative behavior, violence, unhealthy subservience, misuse of power, fuzzy decision-making, false sense of weakness, chauvinistic behavior, and so forth. It is true that on a wide scale these tendencies cry out for historical or economic explanations, but perhaps they arise from a common, very primal, cause.

If we are doing this to ourselves then we can change it. True, biology has encoded us for certain behavior, but it is possible to install new software. What if we all learned to make love without this haunting sense of deprivation? Imagine the enormous potential that lies in mastering an inner state of abundance and vitality instead. Generosity, the flexibility to try new approaches, and a balanced perspective about how to employ resources would become as natural as the shortsighted greed and power struggles that now plague us. When we learn to outwit biology we will reflect back to ourselves a fundamentally altered society.

Summary

- It is possible to get around the biological impulse to engage in fertilization behavior *without* severe frustration.

- We consciously associate passion with pleasure, but our subconscious associates passion with death. This creates defensiveness between intimate partners.

- Conventional sex leaves us with a sense of deprivation that makes relationships draining.

- Mutual giving is the best way to create a sense of safety and abundance, and to heal the typical subconscious uneasiness associated with intimacy.

Nicole's Story

I got serious about learning to make love without orgasm long before I found your material. I read a Tantra book that said women sometimes unconsciously engage in power plays by pushing their partners to ejaculate. And I have to say that I always got a thrill out of my partner's surrender in the throes of orgasm. I realize that men are subconsciously programmed to "spread it around," but I think we're programmed to "pull it out of them."

Before we met, one of my lovers had been in an ashram (celibate) for years. I couldn't help noticing his severe depression several days after we would make love. I'd begun to wonder if I was doing him a favor.

While I was struggling with this inner conflict I got a clear message that passion was a bad idea. A friend brought an attractive man to a party at my home. In our conversation he told me all about his creative work. Lars was a gifted graphic designer, sensitive, sincere, courteous, and somewhat shy. He was accompanied by a polite but much older woman, with whom I didn't speak much. I didn't realize they were lovers. A few weeks later the friend who had brought them both to my house showed up again. He was shattered; Lars was dead.

Apparently Lars had only been with the woman a few

months. And during that time he'd had periods of utterly uncharacteristic, violent behavior. For example, he got into fights in bars and had even been threatened with arrest. My friend, who had known Lars' whole family for years, also talked with his lover after Lars' death. She told him Lars had become sexually aggressive. The night of his death his lover had refused to participate. She went into another room to lie down. He came in later, sat on top of her, and demanded that she make love. She said, "No." He pulled a gun from behind his back and shot himself in the head.

Now, it's *possible* that there was no link whatsoever between his emotional/behavioral deterioration and his sex life. It was clear to me, though, that some sort of severe imbalance certainly corresponded with the period of their intimacy. I promised myself to stop using my sexiness to put others at risk.

Chapter 6

The Spread of the Separation Virus

ON A RECENT VISIT TO NUREMBERG, MY GERMAN HOST
insisted we brave the chilly July rain to look at The Marriage Carousel,
Jürgen Weber's fountain in the heart of the city. The fountain is a vivid
look at the ups and downs of marriage, inspired by a poem written
some four hundred years ago by famous Nürnberger, Hans Sachs. As
you walk around the fountain you see a couple go from their honeymoon in a swan boat through various stages of disharmony. It con-
cludes with a comic look at them still grappling with each other in
hell. Here are selected lines from the poem, which paint a poignant
picture:

... How often during our 33 years of married life
Were sweet and sour flavors
Mixed with happiness and suffering
First up, then down. . . .
My wife is the heaven of my soul,
But also often my pain and hell.
She is my freedom and my choice,
And often my prison and cause of nostalgia ...
My wife is often amenable and good;

She is also often angry and furious.
She is my bliss and my heavy load.
She is my wound and my bandage.
She is my heart's delight
And she makes me old and gray.

Four hundred years later his sentiments still resonate, and certainly women could pen equally colorful lines about their men. True, we can now have casual sex without disgrace and leave each other when heartache strikes. Departure, however, usually buys us a ride on the same carousel with our next lover. Whatever was not working in intimate relationships in the poet's day still is not working.

In fact, as the sexual revolution frees up impulsive sexual activity across the globe, emotional separation between couples is becoming an ever more virulent force. Among other things, it is accelerating the breakdown of the insular family unit. For now, most of us blame the churning in relationships solely on other things, such as readily available birth control, women working and/or collecting child support, easier divorce procedures, and more lenient religious attitudes.

> Sometimes I need what only you can provide—your absence.
>
> —Ashleigh Brilliant

These changes, however, do not account for the urge to separate itself. They merely make it easier for couples to split apart or never commit. Something is stirring up an inability to stay together—and it is ripping apart even the most staid households. Much of this book has been devoted to explaining the physiology behind this urge to separate, but you may still believe, as I once did, that this separation virus infects only a few. Actually it is widespread.

The Bermuda Triangle of Relationships

Not only did Charles and Di split up (despite unlimited checking accounts and an enviable real estate portfolio), even the best matches all too often find their way into a mysterious Bermuda Triangle. Regardless of all efforts to stay on course, many healthy unions between partners who are wise and loving, who communicate well, and who are quite at ease with their sexuality give way to a relentless force. I used to listen to the castaways trying to understand the patterns behind their individual experiences. Gradually, however, I realized that something larger, and quite impersonal, is at work.

It cannot be overcome with good communication or even superior compatibility. Why? Because this pathology is linked to sexual intimacy, which is obviously an integral part of any healthy union. As long-time marriage counselor and author Willard F. Harley, Jr., said in his recent book, *Love Busters:*

> I want to emphasize that [the utter selfishness that so often splits couples up] is normal in marriage. You might think you're married to a crazy person or you may think you're crazy. . . .
>
> I'm thoroughly convinced that it's marriage itself, or more specifically a romantic relationship, that makes communication so difficult. It's not the differences between men and women. . . . [Those I counsel] have very little trouble resolving conflicts when not in romantic relationship.[73]

After years of careful observation, I reluctantly reached the same conclusion. Relationships with sex in them clearly suffer from a baffling fragility. I call it a "virus" because it subverts a healthy element of union—intimacy—and transforms it into a means of damaging the host relationship.

Once I realized that sexual intimacy was somehow at, or near, the root of the problem, I focused more and more attention on happy marriages. How were others managing to evade this insidious force? The closer I examined the successes, however, the more evidence I found of gaps in them. True, in the happiest marriages, the partners were somewhat content with the compromises they had constructed. Upon careful inspection, though, the separation between the lovers was still quite evident. Instead of exhibiting immunity to the separation virus, they established that the malady was more universal than I had first imagined.

As I listened to couples and reflected upon my own two marriages,

A man is incomplete until he is married . . . . Then he is finished.

I grudgingly found myself devising a simple tool for pinpointing where the separation lay in unions. I nicknamed it *The Bermuda Triangle of Relationships* because once conventional sex enters a relationship between committed, sexually compatible partners who sleep in the same place, separation creeps into at least one of these three vital aspects of a healthy relationship: (1) the sexual attraction between the partners fades, (2) they become unavailable to each other sexually even though there is still an attraction between them, or (3) the couple's monogamous commitment breaks or never forms. And without these three cornerstones, the relationship is usually badly crippled, even if it does not die.

Let us look at these three elements in more detail so you will be able to determine for yourself if your favorite fairytale couple has, in fact, beaten the separation virus:

Sexual Attraction

Lack of sexual desire is the most common problem clients bring to sex therapists. I know of a couple so harmonious that they were the envy of their friends for years. Then they shocked everyone by divorcing on the theory that something must be terribly wrong because they were not ever having sex, though they still loved cuddling. Their experience is certainly not unique. According to Oprah's protégé, Dr. Phil, sexless marriages are "an undeniable epidemic."[74]

"I've had to quit making love with my husband entirely," confessed an English friend in a small study group I often attended while in Belgium. "I found it always set off days of inexplicable depression." Moved by her admission, a German friend told us, "After sex I used to get up and go into the bathroom and sit on the tub and cry. I could not imagine what was wrong with me. I had a nice husband, two wonderful kids, and all the money I needed." A third (Danish) was also virtually sexually estranged from her husband and *somewhat* comforted to know the others were sleeping in separate bedrooms from their spouses, too. All were attractive, otherwise compatibly married, and quite comfortable with bodywork, intimacy, and alternative therapies.

Yet all of them opted to "let sleeping husbands lie" rather than try a new approach to lovemaking. One made a brief experiment first. She asked her husband if he would make love without conventional orgasm. After months of weighing involuntary celibacy against "crazy ideas," he agreed. They tried it once, without the suggested gradual exchange of energy over the preceding weeks. "The next day," she told me, "we were like teens in love. We took a walk in the woods. He even lifted me over a fence that unexpectedly barred our way. We giggled the whole way back to the hotel."

The results, though encouraging, were short-lived. The next time they made love, he begged to ejaculate because it was his birthday, and she acquiesced. Within days he seemed to age ten years. "I just can't stand the thought of touching him," she confided. Years later, their unresolved emotional and sexual distance is still a bitter drain on both.

Of course, such decreases in libido are no mystery once you comprehend how conventional sex causes us to associate loving contact with distress, subconsciously or otherwise. Our Intimacy Sabotaging Device (subconscious urge to separate) is just protecting us.

Sexual Availability

The subtlest way partners separate is by becoming unavailable to each other sexually even though there is still an obvious spark between them. The reasons for the separation often appear to be beyond their control. This gap may take the form of incompatible sleeping habits, professional needs to live in different locations, snoring, children's demands, television or reading addictions, illnesses, inexplicable fatigue, sexual dysfunction, obsession with activities one's mate does not share, solo spiritual aspirations, and so on.

"I work fifty to sixty billable hours each week," explained a male friend. "My career has to be my first priority ... at least until I find out if I'm asked to become a partner in my firm. Meanwhile, I just don't have the time or energy to make love much. Between the long hours and my commute, I'm exhausted. My wife and I usually have to go away on vacation to make love, and that isn't easy since she's also a professional. Besides, it seems like every time we plan a trip, some crisis at one of our offices makes it impossible to go—or one of the kids gets sick."

Most of us blame our lack of libido on fatigue, but I now suspect that exhausting ourselves is actually just one more way of avoiding sex. In fact, *For Women Only* by Jennifer Berman and Laura Berman lists various techniques that married women use to avoid sex, from the age-old strategy of feigning sleep to the quite modern practice of taking on household night-owl projects. And women are not alone.

Substance abuse is another common way that couples keep a distance sexually. With alcohol or marijuana, many drift in a haze of pseudo-intimacy for years. From the outside their empty marriages often look all right.

Commitment

This is the most overt way that couples separate. The relationship falls apart, or the partners opt for an open marriage, which usually leads to emotional separation even if they stay together. We have already seen how the hangover from conventional sex weakens a monogamous commitment. When the perception shift hits and your partner looks crazy or selfish, anyone else looks better (the grass-is-greener syndrome).

"I lived with my boyfriend for quite a while before we got married in college," confessed a girlfriend. "We were nuts about each other and very sexually active. The relationship was good for us both. In fact, our grades noticeably improved. But shortly after we married he began to pull away from me sexually. He couldn't explain why, and I couldn't bear the pain of knowing that something was clearly wrong between me and my closest companion with no way to understand it or resolve it. I had an affair with a fellow student. That soothed my wounded feelings, but it made me feel horrible. I'd always prided myself on being honest and genuine, and yet my actions were totally the opposite. But it seemed like losing that sense of closeness with my husband made me feel so desperate that I had very little choice."

Whether or not anyone cheats, emotional disharmony makes ongoing commitment problematic. Someone opts for the noble-sounding ideal of needing more personal space, or both decide they are growing in different directions. Is this problem widespread? In 2002, the Census Bureau predicted that half of all recent marriages will end in divorce.[75]

So this is my Bermuda Triangle. The next time you spot a happy,

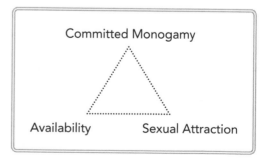

long-term relationship with conventional sex in it, put it to my test. Hold it up against this model. Ask questions to check for gaps in the relationship. If the couple is open and honest, I doubt you will find your test case is the exception to the rule. Relationships with conventional sex develop symptoms of separation in one of these three areas.

"Make love, not war." Hell, do both, get married!

Do not misunderstand me. Healthy relationships *need* these three elements. You cannot have a healing sexual relationship without them. That is why we wisely strive to set up our initial unions around these three cornerstones. However, even these three solid footings are not strong enough to withstand the unfortunate behaviors that, according to the experts themselves, normally accompany conventional sexual relationships. This is why, despite my initial resistance, I have gradually concluded that we have to avoid the separation virus altogether by making love differently. Otherwise biology's mindless insistence on fertilization-driven sex weakens our relationships, or causes them to mutate into disappointing compromises.

Why Isn't *Monogamy* the Problem?

Most of us accept that our hearts open best in an exclusive relationship. I visited a community in Germany, though, whose founders viewed monogamy strictly as an outdated, artificial, economic arrangement between men and women. They condone simultaneous liaisons with partners as a welcome historical correction. Feelings of jealousy or resentment are highly censored.

For years they also held workshops to help people explore their sexuality fully and even set up an erotic academy. One told me that they halted that line of development when too many people became ill after the workshops. Incidentally, the women of the community have an unusually high incidence of pelvic inflammatory disease.

In recent years the community has taken a more spiritual path, seeking inspiration that extends beyond historical logic. And the core members of the community have moved toward depth of intimate connection and away from casual quantity. Indeed, a number of them are now monogamous by choice.

I enjoyed the sense of brother/sisterhood that open intimacy engendered among community members, but polyamory (many lovers) appeared to be a dead-end except when it led to finding a monogamous relationship in which to explore deeper union. If you know your partner is as likely to sleep with someone else tomorrow as he/she is to be with you, there is a level at which you do not surrender. You keep things friendly, affectionate, and sexy perhaps, but you defend your heart a bit. Of course, Romance Junkies are often drawn to such environments because intense experiences are possible and it is perfectly acceptable to drop each partner as your post-orgasmic hangovers catch up with you.

Fairytale Marriages Under the Microscope

Popular wisdom has it that harmonious romantic relationships usually thrive for a honeymoon period of a year or less. To cope with this reality many of us adjust our expectations downward. With the help of trained professionals, we redefine happy relationships as those that stay together though they show significant degrees of stress, emotional separation, and deadening compromise. We are advised to manage these healthy relationships with better communication, endless negotiation, or even gross manipulation. Yet we are not addressing the virus that brings our honeymoons to an end and does us the most damage in the process.

In 2000, Dr. Kiecolt-Glaser released results from a survey of ninety newlywed couples that ran from 1988 through 1992 at Ohio State University. It confirmed the clout of the honeymoon syndrome and measured some of its effects on our well-being. Only couples who seemed to have everything going for them with no addictions or emotional disorders participated. So fewer than five percent of the applicants were selected from more than 2,200 couples. On average they were well-educated and enjoyed annual incomes of $43,000. Most had dated for about three years before they married, and three out of five had lived together before marrying. "These were highly healthy people. They were blissful!" explained one of the researchers.

By the second year of the study, the newlyweds' marital satisfaction had dropped significantly. As Kiecolt-Glaser put it, "Declines in marital satisfaction appear to be a stable response to the first year or two of marriage."[76] By release of the study a fifth had already divorced.

The study had an interesting objective: measuring stress hormones related to marital conflict. During the initial tests the couples were asked to discuss an area of conflict in their marriage for half an hour. Blood samples were taken before and after. Sure enough, hostility had increased the levels of three stress hormones. Regardless of the couples' apparent harmony, these hormones were consistently and significantly elevated in those who later divorced, and remained elevated hours after the discussion of marital problems, even while they slept.

Her Side of the Story: He was in an odd mood Monday night when we met at a bar for a drink. I'd spent the afternoon shopping and I thought it might have been my fault because I was a bit later than I promised, but he didn't say anything much about it. The conversation was very slow going so I thought we should go off somewhere more intimate so we could talk more privately. But at the restaurant he was STILL acting a bit funny. I tried to cheer him up and started to wonder whether it was me or something else. I asked him if it was me, and he said "no." But I wasn't really sure. So anyway, on the way back home, I said that I loved him deeply and he just put his arm around me. I didn't know what the hell that meant because he didn't say it back or anything. I wondered if he was going to leave me! At home I tried to get him to talk but just he got another beer and switched on the television. Reluctantly, I said I was going to bed. Then after about ten minutes, he joined me and to my surprise, we made love. But, he still seemed really distracted, so afterwards I wanted to confront him. Instead I cried myself to sleep. I just don't know what to do anymore. I mean, I really think he's seeing someone else.

His Side of the Story: Lakers lost. Got laid though.

This *His and Hers* joke is also aligned with the findings from the study. The increase in level of stress hormones was greater in women and was a better predictor of divorce than conflict behavior (that is, aggression or negative attitude) during the couples' initial discussions. Notice Her irrational insecurities and fears, projections onto him of her distressed state of mind, unhealthy preoccupation with his perceptions, tardiness, and sense of lack (shopping). Also, notice His puzzling flatness of mood, inability to relate except on a physical, sexual level, communication blackout, alcohol consumption, and total insensitivity to his partner's state of mind.

These symptoms, which are universal enough to make the joke funny, just happen to be typical hangover symptoms following conventional sex. Women tend to become clingy and over-react when the hangover strikes, while men tend to withdraw into their caves and numb themselves with sports and/or substances.

And, as Kiecolt-Glaser said, "These data may underestimate the actual physiological impact of marital discord, since the couples ... were generally quite happy. In other work from our lab we have found that stress can alter responses to vaccines and slow wound healing. Thus, chronically abrasive marital relationships could have important health consequences." Not surprisingly, a Swedish study found that marital stress worsens the prognosis for women with coronary heart disease (while work stress does not).[77] As James Coyne, M.D. said about his recent study on the effects of marital quality on recovery from congestive heart failure, "While a good marriage can give a person a reason to fight their way back to health, a bad marriage can be worse for a patient than no marriage at all."[78] Heart patients who were negative with their spouses were almost twice as likely to die within four years as those who were less negative. The separation virus is hardly innocuous.

Obviously, it is not marriage, but rather harmonious union that helps us. And the wrenching experience of watching our relationships dissolve in mutual stress or emotional distance is bad for us. Another study found that even individuals who were currently married but had been through a broken marriage, were at significantly higher mortality risk compared with consistently married individuals.[79] Perhaps despair sets in more easily for those who have already experienced this virus in their lives.

Tough Call
Research at Yale University indicates that a married man who smokes more than a pack a day can be expected to live as long as a divorced man who does not smoke. As a researcher explained, "If a man's marriage is driving him to heavy smoking, he has a delicate statistical decision to make."[80]

Is the Situation Getting Worse?

Recently I picked up a book by two male psychologist authors who had considered naming it, *Women Are from Earth, Men Are from Uranus*. In fact they named it, *Let's Face It, Men Are \@$$H%c$! What Women Can Do About It*.[81] It was full of brutal advice for coping with abusive men who control intimate relationships with tactics like knowing-it-all, emotional distance, perpetual teenage behavior, or seductiveness. And, no doubt, men could justify a book entitled, *Let's Face It, Women Are Bit*#\%$*, given the verbal abuse and psychological torment they so often engage in while suffering the after-effects of primitive brain programming.

The authors admitted that their goal was not to heal relationships, because, based on their experience, men do not want to change. Instead the authors recommended coping strategies that included burning dinner, parking your partner in, out-silencing him, spending more and more time away from home, and dumping the two-timing charmers. It was entertaining, but it would have been very depressing had my own experience not convinced me that even relationships with these hopeless cases rapidly show signs of good health when they employ a new approach to sex. Meanwhile, many people have, indeed, reached the point of desperation. A gap is widening between the sexes.

My mom said the only reason men are alive is for lawn care and vehicle maintenance.
—Tim Allen

It is not just an emotional gap, either. In a United States Census report for 1996, divorced and never-married people, combined, accounted for forty percent of all adults, up from twenty-eight percent only twenty-six years earlier.[82] And, as I said, nearly half of recent first marriages are predicted to end in divorce, and they are most susceptible to divorce in their early years.[83] In short, committed union is not faring well, though a lot of casual sex is going on. The United States, for example, has one of the highest rates of sexually transmitted disease in the industrialized world.

Until recently, across the globe, church (or social sanction) and state kept a rein on sexual expression. Marriages were often arranged. Divorce was first impossible and then heavily censored. Birth control was unavailable or prohibited. And unsanctioned relationships were strictly punished. All these features of life ensured that any emotional separation between partners was partly masked by the fact that they had to continue to live together. But these circumstances also meant there was just plain less fooling around after the honeymoon period. That left relationships stagnant but less volatile.

Another's wife is a white swan, and ours is bitter wormwood.
—Russian proverb

These rules served the purposes of church and state—institutions that often profited from stable family units preoccupied with procreation. Even now, despite increasing resistance, the Catholic Church is gamely trying to multiply the faithful by encouraging procreation at every turn. And not long ago I came across this headline, "Sri Lankans Urged to Multiply for War." The article reported that the Sri Lankan Government is urging people to abandon the Small is Beautiful birth control campaign and have larger families. Why? To swell the ranks of the army and the clergy. For the same reason, Mussolini ordered the church bells rung in the middle of the night so Italians would wake up and make babies.

I am glad the sexual revolution is helping us squirm free of the short-sighted grasp of such institutions, and I believe the transformation we are witnessing offers great promise for the future. But at the moment things are undeniably ugly. The increased pursuit of sex for the sake of overheated brain chemistry makes messes—unplanned pregnancies, churning relationships, stressed single parents, addicts, miserable kids, and despair about intimacy.

The good news is that our circumstances are so painful that many of us may soon be open to a radically different approach to lovemaking. When we master it the rewards will outweigh the heartache it has cost us to motivate our leap to a new level.

Some of us may already be pointed in the right direction. Undaunted by the grim statistics, people age 20 to 29 apparently hold a more exalted concept of marriage than the centuries-old (but once revolutionary) ideal of friendship in marriage. In a recent Gallup poll of more than a thousand young people, an overwhelming majority were seeking, and expected to find, a marriage that was a spiritualized union of souls. Three-fourths of those polled also agreed that if they met a person with whom they could have a long-term relationship, they would try to postpone sex until they really knew each other.[84] Unfortunately, mere delay may not inoculate them against the separation virus.

Lament of A Great Lover
Q: I love her, and the last time we made love she had four
orgasms. Why would she leave me?

A: There is unfortunately no right way to do the wrong thing.

A New Point of View

One coming gift is the ease with which we can regain our faith in humanity and forgive our past partners as we learn to use sexual relationships to heal each other. It is highly therapeutic to realize that the relationship craziness and chaos we have endured had little to do with humanity's hopeless flaws, different planetary origins of the sexes, our personalities . . . or mental health. Instead we innocently made ourselves nuts trying to please ourselves, or each other, in bed.

Instead of getting married again, I'm going to find a woman I don't like and give her a house.
—Lewis Grizzard

Frankly, this realization already gives my past relationship tragedies a decidedly comic gloss. I now regard our genes and their blind drive to duplicate us as a sort of cosmic prank—one that we no longer need to fall for. Those of us who have behaved the worst while trying to figure out what the heck to do with all of our sexual energy may, in fact, now be poised to spring into the lead in the discovery of true harmony. We are more motivated to transform than those who are stuck in a less acutely uncomfortable stagnation.

As I have started to think in larger terms, the ramifications of our current sex habits increasingly intrigue me. I wonder how many inmates could have avoided lives of crime, addiction, or insanity simply by having a clearer understanding of how to manage their sexual energy. Perhaps many such people are just particularly sensitive to our unsuspected sexual hangover. I wonder whether puberty could become a less traumatic experience if we knew better how to guide our offspring into safe, healthy contact with the opposite sex . . . and themselves.

> Eighty percent of married men cheat in America. The rest cheat in Europe.
> —Jackie Mason

I have even started to suspect that cultural stereotypes develop quite innocently depending upon the accepted role of sex in a given milieu. I notice that sex-positive cultures, like the West Indies or parts of California, tend toward a more playful, relaxed approach to life, along with careless pregnancies, addiction, and unrealistic thinking. In contrast, more sexually repressed cultures, like some of Western Europe and its even more extreme New World descendants, tend toward emotional isolation, rigid, judgmental thinking, and a more responsible outlook.

I think it will turn out that the unhealthy aspects of these extremes will naturally melt away as we replace our inner sense that something is missing with frequent, satisfying union and the inner balance it creates. German psychiatrist Wilhelm Reich argued that dammed-up sexual energy caused all social and personal ills. I think he was onto something. But whereas he seemed to believe that release of sexual energy was the solution, the clues I have seen point to the exchange of sexual energy via the heart as the key.

The energy does have to move for us to feel fulfilled, but it does not have to move in the form of a genital orgasm. Instead it can move in a relaxed, shared ecstasy that gives us a lasting sense of well-being. Reich, after all, was a cocaine addict who married three times, so his emphasis on orgasm could well have hurt him, whether or not it unblocked something.

In any event, as appalling as humanity's current sexual intimacy labor pains are, I am looking forward to what the future holds as we learn to navigate around this weak point in our design, and to chart our course away from biology's nasty Bermuda Triangle for relationships. Instead of lowering our standards for intimate relationships to align with the ravages of the separation virus, let us try raising them substantially to the level of mutual healing. What have we got to lose?

Summary

- ⮞ Committed intimacy is not faring well. Divorce rates are high and the percentage of people who never marry is rising sharply.
- ⮞ The problem is clearly connected with sexual intimacy in committed relationships, but avoiding commitment does not solve the problem.
- ⮞ Separation may show up in any facet of the relationship: broken commitment, lack of sexual attraction, or lack of opportunity to make love.
- ⮞ It is easy to forgive past relationship hurts once we understand the true cause of our dismal results.

Joshua's Story

I was celibate while I attended a six-month training program in California. When it ended I decided to travel before returning to Amsterdam. One of my first stops was a gay beach where I had sex. I was amazed at the depth of the depression that followed within days. It made me think back to the times when I visited such beaches regularly in Holland. I was always sick. Maybe some people aren't affected by it, but sex the way I've been using it does create a hangover for me.

My path of personal growth has been to acknowledge my true worth and deepest desires. As I've moved toward what I really want, my diet has changed to healthy food, my job has changed to activities I enjoy (I'm training to be an acupuncture therapist), and I am ready to try this approach to sex. Deep inside I know sex was not created to make me feel bad afterward, but to allow me to create union between people regardless of their gender.

Chapter 7

Crossed Wires

While living in Europe I developed a close friend-ship with Mark, a gay American. We spoke almost every day on the phone and shared everything. He was the brother I never had. One day I asked him, "If there were a pill you could take to become straight, would you want to take it?" I was expecting him to say, "Certainly not, I love men." Instead he answered, "Yes, in a heartbeat." When I mentioned Mark's answer to another gay friend he said, "Of course. I would, too." And when I asked him why, he said, "Because I have the sense that my wires are crossed."

Poof! There went my picture of happy homosexuals who were just like me except for a reverse spin on gender orientation. Of course, since those discussions, I have come to realize that I have even more in common with my gay friends than I initially imagined. Indeed, everyone on the planet has a case of crossed wires, thanks to our prim-itive brains. They are just crossed in different ways and some are more colorful than others.

From my revised vantage point there is little difference between promiscuous singles, confused priests, loving lesbians, heterosexuals stuck in emotionally distant marriages, adventurous bi-sexuals, lonely masturbators, or even blander variations on the theme of human sexuality. All are but indicators of a deteriorating dynamic of separation between the sexes. I am confident that no one's attempt to cope is inherently, or morally, superior to any other. And none of them heals the dilemma I am addressing either; biology is still pushing us all around.

Who's Driving?

At the time, I was floored by my friends' candid answers. An image haunted me of people trapped on a bus, with a crazed driver at the wheel, careening down a mountain to some destination they would never have chosen. When I talked to a close lesbian friend about it, she assured me that gay men were *different.* With an air that implied lesbianism represented the next rung of human evolution, Chris explained that she and her friends were more than satisfied with their lot.

I found that easy to believe. By then I had been through the hamburger grinder of heterosexual relationships way too many times, and the concept of a relationship with a close friend of the same sex struck me as eminently sensible. I would not have to explain to her repeatedly how to make me come. I could "PMS" without feeling like a public nuisance. Indeed, I toyed with the idea that *I* was the unhappy prisoner . . . of the sensors in my nose that melt me in the presence of certain male pheromones.

Any thoughts of "reform" were dashed, though, when my lesbian friend, Chris, showed up in tears to stay with me for ten days. Her lover was so addicted to orgasm that if she did not make love to her every night Jen would "accidentally" hit her while she slept. This time the violence had erupted while they were awake. Chris was a battered woman.

I concluded that I might as well stick to men. Obtuse as they often were, at least they never hit me. At the end of Chris' stay I watched with horror as she returned to her unhealthy relationship. And since I had counseled her to leave Jen, she pretty much

The Bible contains six admonishments to homosexuals and 362 admonishments to heterosexuals. That doesn't mean that God doesn't love heterosexuals. It's just that they need more supervision.

—Lynn Lavner

quit talking to me ... except to complain that the elegant Jen was gaining weight, which apparently was not part of their unwritten contract.
At any rate, when I saw them a couple of years later, they had both
aged a lot and begun to smoke.

The Prince and the Frog

But back to Mark. Early on, my friendship with him was
very challenging for me because he sometimes engaged
in unsafe sex in the bushes of a city park. In the midst of an AIDS epidemic it was hard to sit with the fact that someone I dearly loved was
trying to destroy himself. But I accepted that I "was not his mom,"
so, except for paying for his clinic visit to treat a case of gonorrhea, I
remained in the role of confidante. Of course, I also showered him
with lots of advice about the hidden perils of genital orgasm, and we
talked frequently about intimate details.

Mark shared that he masturbated relatively infrequently, as compared with another gay friend who had transformed his second bedroom
into an altar to pornography. But whenever he did, it was soon followed by a devastating loss of self-confidence. Some event, like a discussion with his family members, who were not thrilled about his
bumming around Europe without a career, would unnerve him completely. And that is when he would go off to the bushes feeling worth-
less and searching for a thrill (to raise his dopamine level?).

It took some time to spot the pattern, but he finally quit masturbating. Not only did he then forsake the park shrubbery, but within
a few months he got together with one of his early lovers in New
York City, whom he had lost contact with ten years earlier. Theirs
became Mark's first real relationship. That was definite progress,
though they did sometimes have conventional orgasm, despite my
evangelism. Things were predictably chaotic, too, and they screamed
at each other a lot. Mark was an accomplished mooch, and Eric, an
interior architect, understandably frequently lost his patience with
being manipulated.

About a year into their relationship I moved to New York City. Eric
had just given Mark a tyrannical ultimatum. So Mark and I decided to
apply for jobs at a soon-to-open Barnes & Noble superstore. We started

work at a time when Mark and "Mr. Wonderful" (as Mark called Eric) were estranged. Eric was out of town and Mark was working up the courage to leave him now that he had a job. I stayed at their place because he wanted company and we hung out, laughing and talking, for several weeks.

During those weeks I got a glimpse of a very different Mark. Our employer had a clever strategy for appointing managers. It threw all 450 employees into a four-story building together as equals. Boxes had to be unloaded, moved around, and unpacked, so teams spontaneously formed and leaders appeared. I was dazzled as Mark bloomed into a brilliant natural leader: charismatic, hard-working, funny, reliable, and a genius at kidding slackers into full participation (after all, who knew more than he did about evading work?).

He also crackled with a magnetic, thoroughly masculine electricity I had rarely glimpsed, but which he now wore as naturally as a fairy-tale prince. He flirted with women in ways that melted them all, and everyone, of both sexes, wanted to work with him. It came as little surprise that he was promoted twice in those first two weeks.

Unfortunately he was soon to slip back into his frog costume. The last day before Eric's return, he helped me carry my stuff back to my cramped apartment, and we had a long talk about his relationship blues. I invited him to share my space until he, or we, could find another place to live. He was torn. He was acutely aware that before him was an open gate to a totally different lifestyle, and he, too, was enjoying his transformation. But it was also scary.

When he left panic set in. He went straight to a Times Square porn theater and jerked off. His queeny persona swiftly reappeared. He decided to stay with Mr. Wonderful, "because his apartment was so much nicer." He began to offend people at work with his manipulative gossiping, and it was not long before he quit his job at the bookstore. As he explained, "Eric needs me to help him select *fabric* samples and I just *love* fabrics!" I could not help wondering just how many of the world's great natural leaders are confining their talents to fabric selection.

The Penny Drops

Six months later I, too, left Barnes & Noble, to take a job as Cabaret Room Manager for a gay nightclub in Greenwich Village (owned by a straight friend of mine). For almost a year, I designed posters for drag queens, made more friends, and talked with people about humanity's separation virus. Initially I was amazed at the open-mindedness of my homosexual friends. Then it dawned on me that people drawn to same-sex relationships have probably spent more time wondering about the reasons for alienation between the sexes than anyone but me. Far from being threatened by my ideas, many related easily. In fact, almost all friction surrounding my thoughts about same-sex relationships has come from well-meaning but overeager heterosexual defenders of diversity. Diversity is a nice objective, but if you are trapped on a bus you would not have chosen to board in the first place, it may not be your chief concern.

Anyway, a couple of years later, a friend (whom I had not known was bi-sexual) introduced me to Kate. My friend, who enjoyed drama, had "forgotten" to tell me Kate was homosexual. "On a 1–10 scale of lesbianism, I'm about a 15," Kate told me later. "I've never slept with a man. I can't even stand the thought of it. I love women, though." However, that first evening I missed the signals: the discreet rainbow earring, the black leather jacket, and the defiant glint.

I only saw a brilliant engineer with a remarkable ability to concentrate, a broad-ranging background in spiritual matters, and a powerful will, who asked some of the best questions I had heard. Thus began a lively exchange between two very determined Truth Seekers. Kate and I agreed on a surprising number of major points, including the concept that the split between male and female is the means by which humanity perpetuates its dualistic thinking. Kate did not, however, accept that curing an unwholeness of mind might call for physical union with the other half of our species as a starting point.

"But what if unconditional giving, even to that extreme degree of nurturing, were necessary?" I theorized. "Could you agree to reunite with a man in the role of a planetary healer?" Kate was studying for an additional degree in naturopathy by correspondence, and people often came to her for advice. "You wouldn't say you could only treat women if a man needed help, right?"

"Of course not. I help anyone. I just *enjoy* helping women a lot more," she smirked. "Besides, I've always been invisible to men, except as a colleague."

I countered, "I think your discrimination goes deeper than you think. You forgive women anything while you become completely exasperated with a man who does something you don't like."

Kate got very quiet. "I'll work on it," she said with the grim determination of a true spiritual warrior. A week later, I got an email from one shocked lesbian! Following deep spiritual work on releasing resentments she was harboring toward men, Kate was asked out by a male colleague. The day of their date she suffered a horrible migraine, but the evening was quite a surprise. She ended up telling him all about herself. He only wanted to know if there might be a future together. There was not. She was about to take a job in another state. But several myths had exploded before her eyes. She had realized she did need to heal her feelings toward men. And that as she did she was no longer invisible . . . for better or worse.

Uh oh . . .

To be sure, Kate still had powerful desires to hang out at lesbian bars and websites. But she decided to follow her inner guidance and grudgingly opted for "neutral" . . . just temporarily, you understand. She let her hair grow a bit and did not announce her sexual preference at her new job.

A few months later something had definitely shifted. Men, whom she had previously viewed as thick-witted obstructionists, now fell over themselves opening doors, grinning, offering help, furniture, and information. "And when I wear a skirt they say 'Good Morning' to my legs," she laughed. "Of course, I like women's legs, too. . . ." When I next saw her, she was a different woman. A welcoming smile lit her face where before there had been a defensive impassivity. She laughed more often. She no longer gave off an air of *Kate Against the World.*

She began to hang out with a male colleague with whom she shared a lot of sporting and technical interests. There was no passion or sex, though. "Justin has never even tried to unbutton my shirt," she informed me (smugly). I was puzzled because he sure spent a lot of time with her. Finally she admitted that she had begun masturbating again months earlier. (Shortly after we became friends, Kate had told me that, on orders of her inner guidance, she had given it up during the month before we met, which may have given her the clarity and courage to listen to ideas she would normally have blown off.)

With masturbation back in the picture, the lack of sparks between Justin and her was totally comprehensible. As explained in Chapter 2, masturbation depletes sexual magnetism, though it increases the desire for more orgasm. And it sends out an unspoken message of "I don't need you. I can take care of my sexuality myself." I encouraged her to give it a rest just to test the theory. She struggled for months, perhaps because it was a defense. Finally one of her best friends came to visit for three weeks, which gave her the support she needed to let it go.

As soon as her friend left, Justin began kissing her passionately, and, to her surprise, she even enjoyed it. One thing led to another. Then she let him make love to her "just to see if I [she] could do it without feeling sick." She was so bent on her research that she ignored all my advice about approaching intercourse slowly and consciously and avoiding orgasm. She did not even ask Justin to control himself. "I would have enjoyed a pizza a lot more," she told me after the Big Event, "but at least I didn't freak."

About four days later, however, Justin had a sudden stomach flu, and a few days after that a panic attack while kayaking with her. She was dismayed by his weakness, which endangered both him and the guide who had to rescue him. The following weekend she accepted a date to go hiking with another male colleague. Justin was furious. She was self-righteous. They swiftly grew apart. Shortly thereafter she moved in with the hiker, with whom she still lives. Her career has taken off, and I would like to be able to say that everything is going great between them, but it is not. They have made no effort to avoid conventional sex, and three years later they hardly ever make love, much to her dismay.

Moral of these stories? Forgiveness and avoiding masturbation, while hanging out with a member of the opposite sex, are the keys to uncrossing your wires (that is, the secret to spontaneous magnetism toward the opposite sex). Yet going straight is not the key to relationship harmony; we need to make love differently. I know she will work it all out in her own time. And thanks to her and Mark, I will never again believe the current alienation between male and female is irreversible ... even if someone's chosen defense is sexual preference.

Mystery Revealed?

Of the homosexual friends I have mentioned so far, one is a gifted pianist and conductor, one is a technical genius and a remarkable athlete, and three are fluent in three languages and also excellent musicians. Most have unusually heightened spiritual perception (active third eyes), and many originally wanted to become clergy or pursue spiritual work for the benefit of mankind. Unfortunately, all these talents and high ideals matter little because they cannot make the most of their abilities and lofty aspirations.

The pianist, for example, could be a great composer, if he would find another use for his second bedroom. Kate, the engineer, is like a meteor, in serious danger of burning out from overload (imbalance), and suffering from severe endometriosis (a condition that often necessitates hysterectomy). And the signals from their enhanced spiritual vision, though often remarkably clear, are usually disregarded in the inner storms their urges brew up. This causes severe bouts of self-hatred because their intrinsic standards are high, but, in their judgment, their behavior is often outrageous. In short, they experience an extreme version of what all of us go through while our primitive brains rule.

So when I stumbled upon the following explanation in an esoteric book,[85] it rang true. Unlikely as it may appear, extraordinary abilities, vivid imaginations, and frequent masturbation beginning early in life (a trait they also shared) may all be linked to lofty, but sexist, spiritual aspirations in a past life. Here is how.

> Sex is one of the nine reasons for reincarnation. The other eight are unimportant.
> —Henry Miller

It is well-known in esoteric circles that we can expand our spiritual vision, even without a partner, by re-channeling our sexual energy upward with rigorous self-discipline. Some of us have taken this radical step of forcing open our third eye in past lives. To do it, we chose to cut ourselves off from the opposite sex entirely. (And, given the fallout from conventional sex, we may have welcomed celibacy by that point.)

With our newfound power we not only expanded our awareness but also cultivated exceptional mental, artistic, healing, psychic, or other powers. We could never have developed them had we continued to stagnate in the standard marriage / conventional sex / procreation / support-the-offspring cycle that ensnares most of humanity.

However, this course of action had a hidden drawback. When we strengthen ourselves psychically in one lifetime, we start our next lifetime with an unusually strong flow of life force energy. All this power proves extremely destabilizing, for we arrive with enhanced imaginations, hypersensitivity, and more sexual energy than most. But no instruction manual.

And, of course, we are still not inclined to nurture a member of the opposite sex. After all, we forced our past progress precisely by avoiding them, rather than healing them. When we hit puberty, these factors (loads of sexual energy, ignorance of why and how to manage it, distain for the opposite sex, and fertile imaginations) often combine to addict us to masturbation.

Frequent masturbation, however, causes imbalance, which increases paranoia and a sense of alienation from anyone onto whom we project it. This makes us feel different from others on many levels. Indeed, as Gay Pride Day always colorfully demonstrates, terminal uniqueness reigns supreme in the homosexual community. If we choose a lifestyle that encourages frequent orgasm, our sense of being different virtually entraps us. *Voila!* We are now prisoners on a bus we might well not have boarded had we been able to remember the true significance of, and loftier options for, our sexual energy. This phenomenon of feeling odd as the result of frequent masturbation also affects straight, and undecided, people.

> Man, 60: *I was sure I was bi-sexual all these years. But the results from circulating my sexual energy instead of masturbating have been so dramatic (a sense of direction, an open heart, a desire to connect with others, a new joy in music) that I'm open to another approach. I want to see for myself what this kind of union with a woman can do.*
> —*Jon*

Neurochemical Urges

Biology has a role to play in everyone's crossed wires. For example, *Clinical Neuropharmacology* recently published an article about a man who was given high doses of dopamine to treat Parkinson's disease.[86] Dopamine can alleviate the shaking associated with Parkinson's. After seventy years of uneventful heterosexuality, he suddenly found himself cross-dressing. When doctors decreased his dosage, the urge to put on his deceased wife's clothing evaporated. The researchers hypothesized that excess, or sensitivity to, dopamine may be behind both paraphilias (fetishes) and hypersexuality (sex addictions).

Sexual arousal, of course, can innocently become associated with far more bizarre things than clothing. And for those afflicted it is no laughing matter. A close friend discovered in her late thirties that the torture fantasies that ran in her head whenever she was trying to climax were the product of some insignificant (but apparently painful) genital snipping her pediatrician did when she was a baby. Discovering the cause did not heal the association, however. In fact, she still never came without heart-closing, torture movies running in her head.

Happily, when she began using this alternative approach to lovemaking, the fantasies swiftly receded, never to return. Placing her attention on her partner's well-being instead of her own orgasm was the cure. Most fetishes are linked to the desire to orgasm. As long as that payoff is in view it is very hard to let them go. Once orgasm is no longer the goal, however, they lose their addictive grip.

> *Looking back, I realize that my loves were, in reality, obsessions. They caused me more pain than pleasure. Sometimes I can't distinguish between pain and ecstasy.* —*Henry Miller*

Heart/Genital Splits

Most of this book is about the gap that develops between the hearts of heterosexuals who have joined genitals. So I am lumping spiritual celibates into this chapter on same-sex relationships because they, too, show the reverse pattern of alienation from the opposite sex. That is, they deliberately separate at a genital level.

I have a number of celibate, and aspiring-to-be-celibate, friends. And after years of listening and observing I am convinced that some celibates so dearly love members of the opposite sex (as a part of their love for humanity), and are by nature so gentle, that they simply cannot face the ugly fallout from conventional sex. They are frightened of sex—with good reason, as it turns out.

> If it weren't for pickpockets, I'd have no sex life at all.
> —Rodney Dangerfield

Perhaps they have had to dry the tears of an abandoned parent or watch someone turn abusive under the influence of the separation virus. They sense (or have experienced) that they, too, could do something hurtful if they engaged in conventional sex, and so they do not. They give their love to God, the Earth, or other causes, and they comfort themselves with good deeds, prayer, meditation, medication, or recreational drugs. They are, of course, perfectly positioned to establish sexual relationships that heal once they realize there is a nontoxic approach to intimacy.

I also believe that some homosexuals seek to avoid hurting the opposite sex by selecting a same-sex partner. Same-sex relationships initially feel more comfortable because those of the same gender tend to deal with post-orgasm fallout the same way. It is easier to cope with a sexual hangover if both of you process things to death, or both of you withdraw emotionally.

Though they park their genitals elsewhere, members of these two groups often make deeper heart connections with the opposite sex than most heterosexuals ever attain. That is, ardent heterosexuals who copulate willingly, but cannot create a genuine emotional tie with a partner, are no closer to uncovering the mystery of a healing synergy between the sexes than those who keep a genital distance. However, a split between heart and genitals, whether it is north or south of the waistline, is still a symptom of humankind's separation virus.

Spiritual Celibacy

My friends aspiring to religious celibacy proved far less open-minded about the existence of a separation virus than my homosexual pals. After all, ancient religious traditions abound that revere sexual avoidance of the opposite gender. In fact, those who view sexual desire as a weakness, which is easy enough to do on this planet, give extra points to yogis, monks, nuns, and themselves when they are successfully celibate. So they generally disparaged my suggestion that ascetic traditions might have overlooked the peace of mind attainable through another approach to union.

> *Fear not the flesh nor love it. If you fear it, it will gain mastery over you. If you love it, it will swallow and paralyze you.*
> —*The Gnostic Gospel of Philip*

Their intransigence initially surprised me because celibate traditions clearly affirm the correlation between inner peace and a combination of unconditional love and abstinence from orgasm. So I figured those with serious spiritual practices would be among the first adherents to this ancient alternative, especially in light of the many scandals surrounding gurus and clerics. Clearly we have not found a reliable path to spiritual enlightenment unless it balances sexual desire.

Instead, I was surprised to find that when these friends broke their vows, they did so with abandon. They resisted taking a slow approach to sex and tended to focus on their own sexual gratification. After bingeing, they swiftly returned to their special relationship with God, or the feet of their chosen spiritual master. They would explain, often with distain for anyone who did not share their need to atone, that it was an error to think sex could be anything but a red herring for one on a spiritual path. Then, at their next opportunity they would do it all again, often with a noticeable lack of regard for their erstwhile partners. They even found it difficult to treat their "errors" with compassion, perhaps due to guilt projections. At any rate, the concepts of *sex that is not oriented toward physical gratification* and *selflessness toward an intimate partner* eluded them.

> *True love is a completely pure and unencumbered form of giving.*
> —*Gerald G. Jampolsky*

The friends for whom the bell really went off in response to my hypothesis have been those with earnest spiritual practices, who have also tried celibacy, but generally opted for relationship. They have quickly grasped that sex without orgasm is the obvious way to be in integrity with their spiritual work and at peace with their sexuality.

So if celibacy has not lived up to its promise of peace of mind and a seat at God's right hand, stop fighting yourself and try a more generous approach to a higher end. Remember, if you insist on climbing the mountain alone, your gains may be of little value next time around because your inner balance is not complete. Indeed, unless you have healed all subconscious alienation from the opposite sex and your love is unconditional, you may unwittingly be reserving both a seat on the "hopelessly-driven-by-my-impulses" bus and a costume of the gender you are avoiding (so that you can master compassion for its challenges).

Be Bold

Given the damage inflicted by our primitive brain programming, no attempt to cope is surprising. Many of us have understandably unzipped the zipper between male and female in reaction to our uneasiness. Yet we may have the option of healing the unconscious impetus behind that choice.

So if you are settling for an uncomfortable ride, on a bus you are not driving, to a destination you would not have chosen (or if you just cannot get your bus up the mountain on your own), you may have an unsuspected alternative. You may be able to re-pattern your subconscious by gently *un*doing the past damage your procreation-based programming has unwittingly caused. Whether you are now gay, celibate, straight, or undecided, the damage takes the form of a protective desire for separation from the opposite sex (at some level). Therefore safe, healing union between the sexes most directly replaces the old programming, restoring your free will and offering a fresh start.

The first phase of the *Exchanges* (Chapter 12) does not include intercourse. So if you try them, you will have plenty of time to assess whether or not you do indeed feel a new sense of ease and wholeness before intercourse is even an option. Think about it. It could put you in the driver's seat.

Summary

- Most of us suffer from some degree of alienation from the opposite sex, usually in the form of fear or anger.

- Uneasiness about ongoing intimacy with the opposite sex takes many different forms: dissatisfied celibacy, shallow relationships, homosexuality, stagnant monogamy.
- High dopamine levels appear to be associated with fetishes and sexual addiction.
- Affectionate contact with the opposite sex, combined with avoiding orgasm, seems to help heal alienation from the opposite sex.

The Return Home

Although most people spend their entire lives following
this biological impulse, it is only a tiny portion of our
beings. If we remain obsessed with seeds and eggs, we
are married to the fertile reproductive valley of the Mysterious Mother but not to her immeasurable heart and all-
knowing mind. If you wish to unite with her heart and
mind, you must integrate yin and yang within and refine
their fire upward. . . .

The result [of dual cultivation, in which yin and yang are
directly integrated in the tai chi of sexual intercourse] is
improved health, harmonized emotions, the cessation of
desires and impulses, and, at the highest level, the
transcendent integration of the entire energy body.

—Lao Tzu, *Hua Hu Ching*, third century B.C.

[At last] I understood that Eden was a state of being on
the other side of perception. We were kept out of
paradise not by some Biblical illustrator's sword of
archangelic steel but the sharper blade of the firing of our
neurons. Our very bodies—nerve by nerve and
membrane by membrane—were our state of exile, but
they were also our way back in.

—Richard Grossinger, *New Moon*

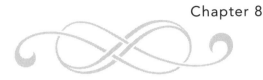

Chapter 8

A Mystery Unfolds

As you have read, recent scientific research supports the conclusion that our physical design leaves us vulnerable to unpleasant side effects from biology's drive to duplicate. The research also suggests that we can escape this fate by consciously changing our body chemistry with altruism, thereby sustaining profound heart connections. Radical as this method of dodging our biological destiny may appear, the most mind-expanding insights related to sacred sexuality are found in various little-known texts. Learning to use sex differently may have implications far beyond relationship harmony, improved health, or even a healed planet. This chapter is for people who enjoy exploring the concept that we are more than flesh and blood.

> In the beginning the universe was created. This has made a lot of people angry and been widely regarded as a bad move.
> —Douglas Adams

You have to admit that, even apart from our crumbling romances, life is no soak in the hot tub. As we tend to see it, we are fragile, often frightened, and dependent upon sperm, labor pains, and morticians to get us through our brief existence. Who wrote this script anyhow? Well, it may turn out we did.

Various sources insist that behind (and concurrent with) the chronicle of biological evolution another epic is unfolding. It is a saga of more numerous and expanded dimensions: the tale of Divinely created beings frolicking throughout a multilevel universe, some of whom chose to wade around in matter. Unfortunately they fell asleep in it for millions of years and, in their uncomfortable confusion, generally blamed their nightmares on a Creator. ("Divine," "God," "Source," "Creator," and "Spirit" will be used interchangeably to refer to the ultimate power behind all of creation.)

How did it happen? By splitting into genders. We take gender as a given, so immersed are we in our particular adventure. Yet gender, if you think about it, is really an uncomfortable longing for wholeness. And it may not be our native state. Edgar Cayce, a highly regarded spiritual healer and seer of the last century, explained that Adam was as androgynous as his Creator until he "projected" himself into an animal body, or rather two. Men were left with a male polarity, while women inherited the female charge. This split dimmed our perception so severely that we forgot how to reverse the process and have been replicating, or rather *recycling* ourselves lifetime after lifetime ever since.

Our electrical imbalance (gender split) accounts for our innate sense of lack. In short, what we think of as normal is actually a handicapped state. Cayce reported that,

> Much might be said respecting the necessity of that union of influences or forces that are divided in the earth in sex. In the heavenly kingdom ye are neither married nor given in marriage; neither is there any such thing as sex; ye become as one—in the union of that from which, of which, ye have been a portion from the beginning.[87]

And stabilizing our relationships to bring these opposing forces (male and female) back into dynamic balance may also be a way of realigning with the oneness of Spirit. In other words, when we employ our sexual attraction to rebuild an unshakeable sense of wholeness or completion it can restore our innate spiritual vision, enabling us to find the way out of our material-plane maze.

Why did we choose to experience ourselves as split into two genders? Apparently it was the lure of erotic arts and crafts. That is, the biological mating game looked like fun. But it was also the way we "fell" into matter, according to another seer of the last century, Harold Percival. He tells us that Adam and Eve were once linked by a sort of psychic cord. Feeling complete, they did not even have a concept of "other" and existed in a state of grace, immortal and free of all anxiety. When they chose to play the mating game, though, the oneness between them rapidly dissolved and their experience changed radically:

> The use of the procreative power was the "original sin." The result following the procreative act was to give to the human race the tendency to unlawful procreation; and this tendency was one of the means of bringing on ignorance and death in the world.
>
> Now [humans are] dominated by that which they originally refused to govern [the sexual urge]. When they could govern they would not; now that they would govern, they cannot. One proof of that ancient [error] is present with every human in the sorrow that follows an act of mad desire which, even against his reason, he is driven to commit....[88]

In fact, we still possess the ability to govern ourselves (and restore this vital link that allows us to feel whole), but it does take patience and determination to overcome our fertilization-driven sexual programming. And it is perhaps significant that the mechanism necessary to achieve it calls for a use of sex that is totally inconsistent with the use of sex for procreation (i.e., no genital orgasm). As an amateur spiritual archeologist, I also find it intriguing that the devil is traditionally pictured as half animal and the grinning captor of a man and woman chained apart from each other.

Male: Hey, Baby, how do you like your eggs in the morning?

Female: Unfertilized.

Like most people, I sincerely wanted to believe that humanity's ideal was an insular family, cemented around a happy couple, with the primary objective of procreating in stability. I adored and married my first lover and would have been pleased had my relationship history ended there. But this ideal may be more and more difficult to sustain as we awaken from our lengthy experiment in animal husbandry. And messy as things look at the moment, the chaos may indicate that Spirit is at work with a very lofty goal: rescuing some fallen angels—us.

The Trap of Duality

Numerous great spiritual traditions teach that matter is a sort of three-dimensional illusion. By that they mean that there is a greater reality behind our experience to which most of us are blind. That larger reality is not bound by our familiar limitations, such as time, space, death, or birth.

Apparently our bold foray into matter has (temporarily) cost us our ability to experience that larger realm. That is, a multidimensional reality of exploding creativity still envelops us, but we think and see in much smaller terms. We are like Truman in the movie *The Truman Show*. We inhabit a bubble in a particular dimension, and we assume it is the whole ball of wax . . . until we are willing to take the necessary steps to restore our full range.

The Bible says that a deep sleep fell upon Adam, and nowhere is there reference to his waking up. —A Course in Miracles

---

It may be that our invisible fence is constructed of a gender split, uneasiness, and our resulting narrowed perception. Certainly, gender leaves us feeling not whole, or split. Any feelings of well-being tend to be short-lived, which is very stressful. Our fear then blinds us to our greater reality. How? It is impossible to experience our oneness with the rest of creation while we believe our safety lies in protective emotional isolation. Even a Creator can look scary when we are anxious. As Voltaire once said, "God created man in His image . . . and man returned the favor." No wonder we fabricated human notions like Divine wrath or, heaven forbid, Divine vengeance.

A number of spiritual traditions refer to our spiritual blindness as "dual perception." That term denotes our tendency to feel that we are separate from others . . . and even from our Source. This duality is why we think about almost everything in terms of good (beneficial to us) and bad (harmful to us). It is extremely difficult to overcome our dual perception (and the defensiveness and greed it creates) while gender feeds a sense of uneasiness, or lack. Cravings make us fearful, and when we act on them hangovers worsen the situation.

Remember, there is a way that seemeth right to a man but the end thereof is death. —Edgar Cayce, speaking about selfishness in sex[89]

134

This perennial sensation of deprivation also fuels our endless search for new toys, more money, and greater thrills. It is behind our inability to feel content for long. Our mechanical searching also keeps us from goals that might offer genuine satisfaction, such as finding our life's purpose, hearing our intuition clearly, bonding deeply with another, or gaining insight about God's will that we awaken.

In short, this craving mechanism acts as a sort of spiritual anchor, ensuring that we spend our short lives recycling each other and then running down our batteries with little genuine satisfaction. Unable to sense our larger reality, we cling ever more tightly to matter, its familiar limitations and fleeting delights, our illusions about our circumstances, and, above all, our firm conviction that we would not exist at all if it were not for our (genes') drive to procreate.

Maybe, as the Divine sees things, human existence is *not* an eternal morality play about the progress of pilgrims that glorifies the righteous and punishes those who err as a result of a flawed design we all share. God may care far more about our long-delayed graduation than our report cards, and regard even the most righteous among us as foot-draggers stubbornly hunkered down in matter, idly twiddling various appendages until we choose to reverse engines. Even now our Creator could be scratching His/Her radiant noggin amazed that we forego returning to full power to continue pursuing short-lived physical gratification. I suspect "Go forth and multiply" was only the first part of a command, the remainder of which was, "until you tire of your diversion, kids, and want to regain your sense of oneness with Yours Truly."

[By bringing a child into the world] you continue the cycle of suffering. Aware that having more children in his society would be to make them suffer, the Buddha urged the monks not to have children.[90]   —*Thich Nhat Hanh, Buddhist Monk*

Buddha was right. Millions of people are brought onto the planet under horrific conditions. An Ethiopian once explained to me that because starvation is so common in his country, families produce as many children as they can (often a dozen or so). If they are lucky, *one* will survive to look after his parents in old age. I cringed at the possible karmic repercussions from this perfectly rational plan.

In any case, the illusion of which great spiritual teachers speak appears to be sustained by our physical design, which engenders and exacerbates an often desperate sense of lack. As Buddha taught long ago, all unhappiness is born of desires (over-stimulation of the pleasure/reward mechanism). So are a lot of babies. In fact, those of us most susceptible to such intense cravings no doubt reproduced the most. By mating fast and furiously we have unwittingly been selecting in favor of intense cravings (and ensuing unhappiness) for a very long time. Biology has been strengthening our drive for continuous sex (or its pleasure/reward surrogates like alcohol and drugs). And both our desire for relief and our conviction that we are hopelessly shackled have grown.

For better or worse, there is little likelihood of overcoming this barrier to restored spiritual vision by continuing our current habits. Because of the way our body chemistry operates, it often makes our desires more severe when we yield to them. The repercussions of both excess and abstinence isolate us emotionally. Over time we defeat ourselves from within—unless we learn to use the same means for a different end.

> It is the essential genius of Tantra that the most basic and most powerful of human instincts is used as a skillful means to stimulate, or expand, awareness and create insight into the nature of reality, and to generate the will to selfless service....
>
> There is no trace of hedonistic indulgence [in the Buddhist Tantra] .... The equation of sexual indulgence and the Buddhist Tantra has been formed by misguided, commercially motivated individuals pandering to the prurient neuroses of the sexually jaded.... "Do not be loose with your sexual organs," advised [ancient female Buddha and Tantrika] Tsogyel. "Bind them fast." And "preserve the seed of kindness [sexual essence] for the sake of other beings."[91]

Toward Better Vision

Long ago, Chinese Taoist master Lao Tzu put it this way: "The cords of passion and desire weave a binding net around you." Therefore the great spiritual traditions advise us to channel our desire toward goals that cannot hurt us: desire for inner peace, desire for wholeness, desire to love unconditionally, desire to experience our fundamental oneness with each other, desire for union with the Divine. Movement toward these goals tends to ease our sense of lack. Achieving them may some day reveal that we are not, in fact, chained to matter.

Some of us cosmic tourists, using various spiritual practices, have overcome our spiritual blindness long enough to glimpse the larger reality behind the three-dimensional movie screen on which we usually focus. Because humankind has generally known of only one (very taxing) way to make love, people tend to make the most spiritual progress when they renounce the world *and* opt for celibacy. These conditions often make it easier to maintain the necessary prerequisites for expanded vision: inner peace and open hearts.

> *Refined semen is stored in the heart center as "radiance," which produces long life and gives a shine to the complexion. Unrefined semen is excreted during sexual intercourse and is, of course, procreative seed. . . . Not only is desire vitiated by orgasm, but the will to enlightenment itself is temporarily lost.*
> —*Keith Dowman, Buddhist scholar*

Given our proclivity for biologically-driven sex, devotional celibacy seems like the obvious starting point in any quest for spiritual clarity. Intriguingly, however, there are little-known sources that point to another path. Take, for example, the ancient Tibetan Buddhist myth, *The Great Stupa.*[92] It confirms that passion is indeed the reason for mankind's fallen state, and says there are three paths to liberation:

- ✤ the overcoming of passion through renunciation,
- ✤ the neutralization of passion by pouring all one's energy into selfless service, and
- ✤ the conquering of passion through controlled indulgence. That is, using sex itself in such a way as to transcend passion's treacherous downward suction.

It says that the third path is the fastest and most powerful path, although also the easiest to fall from ... until one masters it.

The myth, which is very old, predicted there would come a time when the unstable energies produced by increased indulgence in passion would create chaos at both seen and unseen levels across the globe. The first two paths, celibacy and compassionate service to others, would no longer open the door to enlightenment, though they would remain useful spiritual disciplines. Why? Because general unrest would render impossible the necessary degree of inner stillness.

Instead only the third path, balance with a partner, would serve. Apparently a loving relationship, devoted entirely to the goal of transcendence, can create enduring inner peace and stability. In this way, we can reconnect the broken circuit of gender and permanently rise above our built-in sense of lack. By contrast, celibacy still allows gender polarity to create severe longings in many of us, if only for simple loving touch. And I suspect this trait is less a product of moral weakness than a result of the easily inflamed body chemistry that we have bred into ourselves for millennia. These bothersome longings may also mask intense yearnings for reunion with our Source. The silver lining? Many of us are apparently now primed for shared enlightenment should we care to use our urges for a higher end.

A survey conducted by the Gallup Organization from January to March 2001, from a statistically representative national sample of 1003 young adults ages twenty to twenty-nine found that:[93]

> Young adults today are searching for a deep emotional and spiritual connection with one person for life. At the same time, the bases for marriage as a religious, economic or parental partnership are receding in importance for many men and women in their twenties. Taken together, the survey findings present a portrait of marriage as emotionally deep and socially shallow. . . . Only 16% of young adults agree that the main purpose of marriage these days is to have children.

"The Ark of Peace is Entered Two by Two"[94]

Another source, *A Course in Miracles*, also declares that relationships are God's plan for restoring us to whole-mindedness.[95] It says that the purpose of relationships is solely "to make happy" and to heal.[96] The false belief that we can create ourselves is the foundation of our illusion, and we attack all efforts to bring it to light.[97] In other words, the entire birth/death gig is part of our illusion. In the eternal now (which seems to us like millions of years still ticking away), we are simply fragmenting ourselves over and over without truly creating new beings. Nor have we ever changed the way God sees us: one, immortal, and whole.

To free our minds from our self-created false perception, we let go of our conceptions of reality and restore our minds to wholeness. According to *A Course in Miracles* we cannot do this until we learn to use our bodies and relationships entirely differently[98] by finding the middle path that lies between renunciation and indulgence.[99] The way we have come (biology's plan) will not serve.[100] *A Course in Miracles* says we can either have freedom of the body (follow our impulses) *or* freedom of the mind, but not both.[101] In other words, we can indulge our urges or master them to heal our split minds.

> I can resist anything but temptation.
> —Oscar Wilde

Incidentally, *A Course in Miracles,* too, teaches that all our woes come from a sense of lack,[102] which it says we project onto others, causing us to separate from them in fear. We have convinced ourselves that the body will only allow limited indulgences in "love," with intervals of hatred in between that make us fearful of love. We believe that this handicap limits our ability to enter into genuine communion with each other.[103] *A Course in Miracles* says the origin of our distress is "primitive" and more a cause for jest than anguish.[104] I believe the word "primitive" is a reference to the pleasure/reward mechanism in our primitive brain. For a very long time this mechanism has led us to blame others for the effects of an internal imbalance that we create ourselves. And it has also kept us thinking as small as ants in an ant farm.

"Understand the undefiled intercourse, for it has great power"[105]

The key concepts in *A Course in Miracles* closely mirror ideas found in certain little-known early Christian texts. In 1945 in Upper Egypt, a collection of fifty-two documents buried around the middle of the fourth century was rediscovered by peasants digging for gold. Known as the Nag Hammadi library, most of them are Gnostic writings. That is, they claim to record "secret knowledge." Some closely resemble Old Testament Scriptures or New Testament gospels. Like *A Course in Miracles,* the Jesus of the Nag Hammadi texts speaks of illusion and enlightenment, not sin and repentance. Instead of coming to save people from sin, Jesus comes as a guide who opens access to spiritual enlightenment through knowledge.

These ancient fragments also speak of God the Father *and* God the Mother, Jesus and Mary Magdalene as the second Adam and Eve, and of the Sacrament of the Bridal Chamber as the mystery or (final) initiation where a Christian transforms into a Christ. The aim is reunion of the male and female elements on Earth to reflect the divine union of the male and female godhead above. The Gnostic goal of "celibacy," according to Andrew Welburn, was not a denial of sexuality, but a resolution of inner energies, a state of wholeness or innocence.[106]

One of the most intriguing Gnostic gospels is the *Gospel of Philip,* which introduces the Sacrament of the Bridal Chamber. Like marriage, it involves a formal commitment between partners. But the key to the sanctity of their joining is a sacrament of sexual union that aims at higher levels of balance, heightened consciousness, limitless energy, and union with the Divine. Its purpose is not physical procreation, but enlightenment. "It is in the bridal chamber, by human action, that the redemption comes about *in this life.*"[107]

The *Gospel of Philip* says that traditional marriage (in which Adam and Eve engaged) is defiled. It transforms spouses into animals who produce animals. The Gospel states, "Great is the mystery of marriage! For without it the world would not have existed. Now the existence of the world depends on man, and the existence of man on marriage. [By contrast] think of the undefiled relationship [sometimes trans-

---

Adam was walking around the Garden of Eden feeling very lonely, so God asked, "What's wrong with you?" Adam replied that he didn't have anyone to talk to.

God said he was going to give him a companion . . . a woman. "This person will cook for you and wash your clothes, she will always agree with every decision you make. She will bear your children, and never ask you to get up in the middle of the night to take care of them. She will not nag you, and will always be the first to admit she was wrong when you've had a disagreement. She will never have a headache, and will freely give you love and passion whenever needed."

Adam asked God, "What will a woman like this cost?"

"An arm and a leg," replied God.

"Well," hesitated Adam, "what could I get for just a rib?"

lated as "undefiled intercourse" as in the heading to this chapter], for it possesses a great power."[108] And, "If there is a hidden quality to the marriage of defilement, how much more is the undefiled marriage a true mystery! It is not fleshly but pure. It belongs not to desire but to the will."[109] Another Gnostic Gospel, the *Gospel of Thomas,* says that Jesus taught:

> When you make the two one, and when you make the inside like the outside and the outside like the inside, and the above like the below, and when you make the male and the female one and the same, so that the male not be male nor the female female . . . then will you enter the Kingdom.[110]

According to Mary Sharpe, researcher at the Faculty of Divinity, Cambridge University, the sexual congress alluded to in these texts is one of contained, undefiled, "immaculate" intercourse. "To all intents and purposes," she explains, "it is the same as the goals of Tantric yoga, Taoist yin-yang equilibrium and the mystical aspirations of the Jewish Kabbalist Zohar. This contrasts with orthodox Christianity, which lays great emphasis on procreation as the purpose of sexual union within marriage."[111]

For the Kabbalist the ultimate sacrament is the sexual act, carefully organized and sustained as the most perfect mystical trance.
—Kenneth Rexroth, author of The Hasidism of Martin Buber

Hmmmm . . .

These hints that there is mystical potential in the union of male and female make me wonder if many of us have been unable to transcend sexual urges despite their attendant woes for a very good reason. Perhaps these urges are, indeed, pointing to The Way Out of our matter-mindedness when we learn to use them to heal our split minds.

While I have not yet achieved the state of united wholeness these sources describe, I can honestly say that every step I have been able to take on this path has led to perceptible benefits. I am unusually optimistic, energetic, and healthy for a woman of forty-nine. My relationship flows with lighthearted humor, mutual support, inspiration, romantic affection, and trust. And whenever I have slipped off my new path, I have been amazed at how those good feelings evaporated (temporarily).

> There is a certain momentary pleasure associated with conventional orgasm, but its effects are psychologically and emotionally degenerative. It constantly reinforces negative emotional states, not the life of love.... As long as the fixation of attention is reinforced pleasurably, and with some consistency, in the lower body, attention will not rise to the higher functional dimensions of the body.... You must find the way of enjoying sexual intimacy whereby life-energy is not lost.[112]

If the unsuspected benefits I have experienced lie hidden in an "ancient new" use of sex, who knows what else might be possible? Indeed, the Alice A. Bailey materials maintain that humankind will go through its first level of spiritual metamorphosis when it learns to transmute its sexual energy from the procreative center up into the higher centers of the body:

Transmutation and Transference
of the Sex Energy

... In that transmutative process men have greatly erred and have approached the subject from two angles:

1. They have sought to stamp out natural desire and have endeavored to emphasize an enforced celibacy; they have thus frequently warped the nature and subjected the "natural man" to rules and regulations which were not of divine intent.

2. They have tried—at the other extreme—to exhaust normal sexual desire by promiscuity, license and perversion, damaging themselves and laying up the basis for trouble for many incarnations ahead....

During the process of evolution ... sex becomes a dominating thought in the consciousness, and many people today are passing through this stage and everybody at some time or in some life passes through it. This is followed by a period of transference wherein the physical pull of sex and the urge to physical creation is not so dominant and the forces begin to be gathered up into the solar plexus ... and gradually are carried up to the throat center, but always *via the heart center.*[113]

I find this material particularly encouraging because it suggests that our widespread distress in intimate relationships could be a signal that many of us are now ready to make a significant leap forward. We have only to learn to channel our sexual energy through our hearts. Apparently we cannot do it either celibate or through exhausting our sexual urge. So the secret to this mystery may be together, with mutual self-control.

What Do We Really Need from Each Other?

Some years ago, a new friend, visibly agitated, asked if he could speak with me confidentially. We walked to the shore and sat on a dune. He was a gifted musician, tall, with a beautiful face, an ethereal, elfin quality, and more than a hint of angst. I wondered if he was going to say that he was gay and struggling with coming out. As we walked I mentally composed a compassionate speech.

I had to laugh at myself when it turned out that his crisis was that he was still a virgin at age twenty-seven. "Gay?" he snorted, "certainly not. I only feel right when I am touching a woman."

That simple statement echoed in my brain for a long time. In those days I was well versed in spiritual self-sufficiency and still censored any suggestion that others could play such a profound role in my contentment. On the other hand, quite honestly, I often felt the same way about men. That is, I did not need any *thing* from them, but I certainly felt better when I was around them, hearing their voices and perspective on things, letting them rib me, hugging them. I knew from experience that I was more balanced, calmer, enlivened, and effective when they were near (except when separation had set into my intimate relationship with one). Weird. As time passed, I also watched homosexual friends visibly relax and brighten up while exchanging non-threatening touch with the opposite sex, such as holding hands or therapeutic massage.

Were we the handicapped few? Or was there a more profound spiritual principle than self-sufficiency? In light of the materials I have laid out in this chapter, I now believe in a powerful synergy between male and female, which is somehow achieved through an unseen energy flow. Perhaps what we most need from each other is simply to complete an electrical circuit of intention to comfort and heal. Unfortunately, however, many of us are still blinded by the things on our ideal-mate lists, like hotter sex, more attractive babies, social status, security, and so forth. These "must haves" are simply projections of our search for inner wholeness. The true gifts of union are both subtler and simpler to attain, once we set our biological agendas aside.

At the level of the body, we will always be separated, at least by skin. So the goal of this other approach to sex is to use our unions to expand our perception until we *experience* our shared identity. I suspect that occurs in the merging of energy fields beyond our bodies. Physical union, and the neurochemical changes that promote bonding and bliss, are thus physical reflections of a subtler union. This may be why selfless caring seems to be more critical to slipping past biology than physical technique. Caring is an intention that directs our energy from our hearts into a circuit with another's energy.

Even though there is still much I long to know about the energetic and esoteric aspects of this path, I am heartened by the fact that we are not seeking new territory, but rather very old territory. Here are some teachings of the ancient Taoist, Lao Tzu, from the third century B.C.:

> A person's approach to sexuality is a sign of his level of evolution. Unevolved persons practice ordinary sexual intercourse. Placing all emphasis upon the sexual organs, they neglect the body's other organs and systems. Whatever physical energy is accumulated is summarily discharged, and the subtle energies are similarly dissipated and disordered. It is a great backward leap. . . .
>
> Where ordinary intercourse is effortful, angelic cultivation is calm, relaxed, quiet, and natural. Where ordinary intercourse unites sex organs with sex organs, angelic cultivation unites spirit with spirit, mind with mind, and every cell of one body with every cell of the other body. Culminating not in dissolution but in integration, it is an opportunity for a man and woman to mutually transform and uplift each other into the realm of bliss and wholeness.[114]

Fleas in a Jar

I once read that if you put fleas in a jar and put the lid on, they will try to jump out. After they hit the lid a few times, though, they adjust the height of their jumps to a level just short of the lid. Then, when you remove the lid, they continue to restrict the height of their jumps to just short of where the lid was. In other words, they will not escape, even though they are free to go.

Biology has successfully convinced us that we are fleas in a jar. Conventional sex causes us to bang ourselves repeatedly on the painful lid of estrangement between lovers. It is no wonder we make choices as stifling as those hopeless fleas did. Maybe we withdraw from relationships altogether, or choose indulgence at enormous emotional and material cost, or settle for deadening, but less draining, relationships.

All are blind alleys. So, like our ancestors, most of us conclude there is no way to express our sexual energy enthusiastically without wreaking havoc. As we shut down, the world begins to look like a very depressing place. Worse yet, an unlimited amount of desperately needed enthusiasm, creativity, and caring are lost to us all.

By allowing biology to lead us around by the genitals, we have unwittingly conspired with it to create the illusion of a prison. I say we find out if there is any truth in these ancient rumors of a transcendental path of relationship. Certainly loving intimacy can be a most potent health enhancement. At its most powerful, though, merging may be like Dorothy's ruby slippers in *The Wizard of Oz*—a means of returning home to wholeness by resolving the blinding discomfort of gender itself.

Why not take the hand of a willing partner and jump as high as you can? At the very least your efforts to find peace between the sheets can make a vital contribution to eradicating the heart-rending virus of separation. And, who knows? There may not *be* a lid on the jar.

Summary

- Biology has created an artificial sense of hopelessness in humankind, which narrows our perception.

- Various esoteric sources suggest that union with another furnishes a path to enlightenment because our native state is wholeness and immortality, not gender and endless birth/death.
- The goal of sacred sex is not procreation, but rather transcendence.
- Avoiding orgasm is as natural as biologically driven sex; it is merely a way of choosing a different destination for our unions.

Part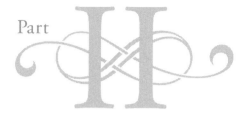

How

All the joy the world contains

has come through wishing happiness for others.

All the misery the world contains

has come through wanting pleasure for oneself.

—Shantideva, ninth century Indian sage

Chapter 9

So You Want to Try It?

I STUMBLED AROUND A GOOD BIT WHILE LEARNING THIS approach to intimacy, and suffered some painful emotional scrapes and bruises as a result. For example, the progress with my soon-to-be husband that could have taken a few short months instead took a year and a half. Mind you, we noticed powerful benefits during that time—gains that were absent in prior relationships with conventional sex. We also learned a lot. In retrospect, however, we suffered much unnecessary heartache, which I sincerely hope you will avoid.

So I heartily advise that you skip all the compromises and gradual integration strategies that will occur to your biologically driven brain, and begin by trying what finally worked, the *Ecstatic Exchanges*. I found that detours, which at the time I genuinely believed were insignificant, always led to long, uncomfortable delays. In this chapter, I have done my best to steer you around my mistakes of the last twelve years.

"We're the Gas, They're the Brakes"

Biology pushes us into certain roles. It forces the man to exploit every possible fertilization opportunity and resist taking "no" for an answer. It leaves the woman in the equally obligatory role of law officer. She must do whatever it takes to keep the man in check unless she wants to have intercourse. This "keep sniffing till she stops growling" dynamic is perfect for dogs, but it will not work if you want to use sex to heal.

Those who documented the existence of the relaxed, valley orgasm thousands of years ago opted for something close to a *reversal* of these roles. As they phrased it, "the woman is the boat and the man is the pilot." The woman's role is to relax into total receptivity, which she obviously cannot do if she has to police her lover. The man's role is an effortless attentiveness, which he cannot deliver if he is blind with impulsive behavior. Ideally, instead of rowing, he merely steers. And it is his function to know exactly where his boat is at all times—that is, the degree to which his partner is aroused—so they can journey safely.

Q: Why are men's brains larger than dogs'?
A: So they don't hump women's legs at cocktail parties.

In addition to this innovative flow of energy, where the woman opens as the man provides a safe space, there are certain other factors that make for safe boating. The key to a man's becoming an infallible pilot rests with the woman. If she is open and loving (rather than seductive), he will find it easy to maintain control. Likewise, the man holds the key to her receptivity. If she knows she is in the hands of a safe pilot she can stop braking completely and fall into a natural state of ecstasy in which he can join.

However, after years of conventional sex, few of us can instantly open our hearts or pilot with absolute safety. The solution to this apparent "chicken or egg" puzzle is time. The *Exchanges,* for example, call for a two-week period where there is lots of snuggling and no intercourse. Time is your friend. You will see progress rapidly, but it takes time to thoroughly master a new practice. So relax and enjoy the re-patterning process.

What to Expect

People are often surprised by the fact that making love this way demands no technical mastery. Instead it requires patience, sustained intimacy, and a willingness to stop the hot (or constant) pursuit of physical gratification. In my experience, authentic love soon flowers between partners in the presence of these ingredients. This is why I advise singles who want to try this to find a partner who is enthusiastic about these *ideas,* rather than someone with whom they are infatuated. Infatuation muddies motives and usually causes someone to bend the rules.

> *Temptation is the dress rehearsal for a karmic experience of negativity.*
> —*Gary Zukov*

For the first few nights of the *Exchanges,* lovers often require special consideration. Those who have been without partners for a while, especially men, can have intense reactions to intimate contact. As one man to whom I described the *Exchanges* told me, "I won't be able to sleep next to a woman; I'll be awake all night." And the fact is, he might. Yet if you both stick with the recipe, this restlessness will pass within a few days.

Some men swing the opposite way. Before they can reach a balanced state of well-being, their mainspring has to unwind. My friend's lover, a dynamic businessman who had been on his own for a long time, spent most of their first few days together simply sleeping—to his chagrin. The advantages of this approach, however, come from achieving an inner balance, so adjustments like temporary restlessness or fatigue are normal. After an initial adjustment, well-being prevails. Even people who slept poorly on their own frequently find that they sleep far better with a partner in this approach to relationship.

So whoever is feeling most centered should willingly put his or her needs aside for a few days. Though it may not feel like it when you are sleep-deprived, your greatest need is for a centered partner. Give him or her "all you can eat" of thoughtful, non-erotic attention. Your generosity will return to you in the form of a balanced, energetic, attentive partner.

It's OK, George

The experience you are now seeking is not dependent upon sustaining an erection. Erections come and go, but the exhilarating exchange of affection on which the rewards of this approach depend is unaffected. This is because a powerful current is actually flowing between your two open hearts.

Intercourse is a reflection of a deep desire to merge, but genitals do not cause desire. Rather, desire reaches ideal levels naturally once all uneasiness is gone. Barry Long, Australian advocate of sacred sex, says that a period of sexual unresponsiveness is natural as we move back into our hearts. It passes when we heal the heart/genital split of the past. So let your genitals show you when this split has healed.

> Sex at age 90 is like trying to shoot pool with a rope.
> —George Burns

Forced performance would merely over-ride any uneasiness about intimacy itself. So it is better to stick to non-performance-oriented, loving contact for weeks, if necessary, to allow your sexual energy to arise spontaneously. Then heart and genitals operate in tandem.

Not-So-Harmless Activities

Once again, this is a different approach to sexual intimacy. The goal is not just intercourse or a dopamine rush of sexual excitement. The goal is the healing that comes from two open hearts. As you may recall from Chapter 4, an open heart promotes the ideal balance of body chemicals, which automatically ensures sexual arousal. In other words, when you have taken a slow approach, and your hearts are truly fear-free, your genitals will be ready. Ready genitals alone do not necessarily indicate open hearts, as our primitive brains can induce performance even while subconscious fear reigns.

A friend suggested I call this book *No Viagra, No K-Y Jelly* because sexual arousal becomes so effortless. The reason it is effortless, though, is that you never force it. Ever. Even if your partner was very aroused last time. Even if your partner would respond rapidly to deliberate stimulation. Just wait … until another occasion. If you follow this simple rule you will find that you hardly ever have to wait. So conventional foreplay, Viagra, vibrators, and anything else that artificially stimulates sexual performance are unwise. Even tongue kissing should wait until after the first few days of the *Exchanges*.

Of course, either partner should feel free to initiate considerate, nurturing touch (as opposed to hungry touch). But, again, if you are a man, never have intercourse unless your partner's genitals are lubricating naturally without physical stimulation, even if she kidnaps your penis. Just rescue it and reassure her with loving affection. She cannot benefit you by having intercourse too soon because, unless her magnet of sexual desire is fully operational, a nourishing current will not flow between you. Forced intercourse, in fact, encourages a heart/genital split.

By the same token, if you are a woman, never initiate intercourse unless your partner has signaled his total enthusiasm and is waiting for you to do the honors. If you indicate that you want intercourse "now," he will do his best to oblige you, even if he is not truly ready. He is likely to force his performance with fantasy or vigorous stimulation. However, his penis will do you no good if his heart is not fully open yet. So wait.

Get a Lollipop

"I'm a very oral person ... and I'm not talkin' about talkin'," said a friend. Sorry, Tiger. Years of experience and frustration have revealed the unwelcome but simple truth: however clear your intentions when you crawl into each other's arms, if you engage in certain activities, your biological auto-pilot will take over. Most people view activities such as dressing in lacy underwear, crawling all over a partner naked, posing nude, frenzied kissing, rubbing genitals on a partner, oral sex, viewing porn, and so forth as harmless. And it seems like they must fit into the picture of healing sexuality somehow.

In fact, they do not fit into the picture of healing sexuality. Innocent and enjoyable as these actions may be, they prevent you from finding the heart-centered ecstasy you are now seeking by pulling all your attention swiftly toward physical gratification of the urge they awaken in your primitive brain. The good news is that with this other approach, intercourse and kissing become increasingly pleasurable. So once you recover from your dopamine rush addiction you will not pine for your former habits. Promise.

> There are a number of mechanical devices which increase sexual arousal, particularly in women. Chief among these is the *Mercedes-Benz 380SL* convertible.
>
> —P. J. O'Rourke

Before leaving the subject of the not-so-harmless, I will share the remarks of another friend. She told me that she did not want to learn this way of making love because she enjoys being such an accomplished lover and she would never get to show off her skills. However, when she left her last boyfriend it was "because I did not want to be f**ked like a porn star." If you want to use sex to heal, dismiss your inner temptress. She attracts equally performance-oriented partners.

To Have All, Give All

Up until now your improved health, career progress, and spiritual goals have seemed to hinge on time spent pursuing them at the expense of other activities. When you create a healing sexual relationship, however, you leave behind the sense of scarcity on which such struggles rest. You plug into a far more effective means of creating balance, well-being, abundance, and heightened spiritual awareness. It is based on giving.

When you give, you program your subconscious for abundance. You convince it that you have enough to give and it begins to react accordingly. Experience it for yourself. While you do the *Exchanges,* make it a point to be extremely generous. Remember, all actions count; so do not measure your devotion in "I love you's," tears of joy, or hours logged in the sack.

Shifting your partner to top priority does not mean that you will have no time for your other activities. In fact, you will swiftly enter a flow that allows you both to accomplish more than ever without having to negotiate at all. But it happens because of inner harmony, which is a product of generously caring for another. So start by voluntarily putting your partner's well-being before your other goals even if you have to break some cherished routines.

A rock-solid relationship is built on knowing you can count on each other—no matter what. If you do not have this security, then no other evidence of love amounts to much. If you do know it, you will find that you want to accommodate each other's interests whenever possible.

No Other Agendas
You can only open your heart fully to someone if you perceive that they have your best interests at heart.

Unfortunately, you may have spent years in draining relationships that caused you to anxiously guard your time and income from your intimate partner. So even if you now understand why you want to give, your giving skills may be a bit rusty. Here are some suggestions to help kick-start your generosity while you try the *Exchanges:*

- Take turns treating each other to things. Splitting is not giving.
- Make gifts to each other. Material gifts are appropriate but nonmaterial gifts of time, energy, and thoughtfulness can be even more healing.
- Treat each other like royalty. For example, never enter a room without checking in with your partner with a smile, a word, or a touch, if possible.
- Be creative spoiling each other with unexpected acts of thoughtfulness:
  - Clean the pan your partner burned the dinner in
  - Suggest an outing or music you know your partner would enjoy
  - Give a spontaneous massage
  - Fill the car with gas even if it is your partner's car, and not your job
  - Put toothpaste on your partner's toothbrush at bedtime
  - Write a mushy poem or note
  - Prepare a favorite dish
  - Leave your partner a surprise treat

When your goal is to pamper another, it makes you feel whole and strong. Nothing is missing. It is the most reliable way to fill the (biologically intensified) empty hole inside that you may have been trying to fill by focusing primarily on your own goals.

Avoid touching your partner when you are coming from a place of hunger. It can make your partner feel like he is being devoured, or like she is stuck nursing a greedy baby. This is a stressful experience. Shift gears and focus on your partner's well-being instead. Nurture your partner, and he or she can nourish you beyond your expectations.

What About Birth Control?

By all means, use it. In theory it only takes one sperm and a friendly egg to bring another being back into matter. In fact, however, it takes a fair number of sperm to penetrate the membrane of an ovum. Some have not used birth control since they began making love without ejaculation years ago, and have not had an unwanted pregnancy. Making love without artificial anything (or worrying about fertility cycles) feels like a visit to the Garden of Eden. Of course, pregnancy without noticeable ejaculation is possible, so take any necessary precautions.

Making love without ejaculation is a true blessing for men. It increases their joint control over the procreation process. The number of viable sperm delivered decreases with the time between ejaculations (after about 48 hours),[115] so with this approach a couple rarely gets pregnant unless both parties agree. Best of all, when we all master healing sex we will not have to listen to the ear-splitting squawks of the "pro-choicers" and "right-to-lifers." Without unwanted pregnancies there is nothing to fight about.

"What If I Have Very Little Sexual Control?"

The *Exchanges* seem to be extremely effective in helping people, especially men, master their sexual energy. For at least two weeks intercourse is not even an option, so you can relax completely and turn your attention to your partner's comfort and healing. You will also feel your partner's attentions more powerfully when you are not driven to get somewhere. This exchange of caring attention balances you both, and balance spells effortless control.

When you enter the intercourse phase of the *Exchanges,* the emphasis will be on motionless, affectionate contact, which also makes control less challenging. Meanwhile, here are some other activities that can strengthen your inner balance:

- Deep forgiveness of all past hurts inflicted by the opposite sex.
- Avoiding masturbation and sexual fantasy, and turning one's attention to helping others instead. (Let your energy flow up through your heart instead of out through your genitals.)
- Preceding intimacy with rigorous exercise, meditation, a warm bath, or a practice such as yoga or tai chi.

Advice for Wilted Plants

Strange to say, one of the traits that can motivate you to reach for higher-quality relationships—that is, your love of excellence—can also be a huge stumbling block. Many of us want to be perfect for each other before we employ the therapy of the *Exchanges*. We want to deny our insecurities, hide our addictions, and live up to some imagined description of each other's perfect mate. This outlook is understandable, but misguided. The only high standard you need to maintain is integrity. That is, stick to the *Exchanges*.

As for your other noble aspirations, it is better if you set out together strictly as you are, with all your current "warts" exposed. This frees your partner to do the same. Warts, after all, are there to be healed, and healing is the sole focus of this approach to sex. So if you have an addiction, a sharp tongue, or a fear of abandonment, admit it. You, like everyone else on this planet, are a wilted plant for the moment. That is okay. Self-doubts are normal. Making love differently will change things for the better, but do not pretend to be something you are not in advance of genuine progress. Each improvement will give you something to celebrate together.

If you have a serious addiction to anything, be optimistic. Many heart-centered people on this planet suffer from addictions. It is a perfectly understandable response to the pain of separation that currently infects us. But addiction is like a mistress. It is a device that sabotages the deep intimacy you are now seeking. So you will not be able to keep your addiction if you want a healing relationship.

If you are clear that you wish to let go of your addiction, the

Exchanges offer superb support. If you cooperate fully by (1) avoiding over-heating and the brain chemistry that accompanies it, and (2) refusing to separate from your lover overnight to pursue your addiction in private, the *Exchanges* will directly heal the isolation (lack of wholeness) that is driving your addiction. With a steady exchange of loving nourishment, you will soon be strong enough to release the unhealthy self-pity that also feeds addiction.

When you begin the *Exchanges,* stop your addiction cold turkey, and follow the instructions exactly. Beware that for a while, a foreign will (born of a past drive to meet your addiction no matter how destructive your actions), may attempt to control you. It will do its best to convince you that you want to cheat on the *Exchanges* and return to passion in your lovemaking, that you are too weak to succeed, or that you should separate from your lover to do your own thing. All are just invalid excuses for resuming your addiction. They do not reflect your true will. Prayer or meditation can strengthen your inner resolve.

And if you fall back into your addiction, do not use it as an excuse to have an orgasm or separate from your lover, too. When you are clear, simply drop your addiction and pick up the *Exchanges* again. Wait to do an *Exchange* until you are free of the direct influence of your addiction, but spend each night together, even if you relapse.

I count him braver who overcomes his desires than him who conquers his enemies; for the hardest victory is the victory over self.
—Aristotle

If your partner is fighting an addiction, accept that he/she must heal it. Your role is merely to hold an unconditionally loving space in which the healing can take place. As long as your partner sticks to the *Exchanges,* be encouraging, forgiving, generous, non-judgmental and affectionate, but stay detached from the outcome. It is not within your control.

NOTE: If you cannot do an *Exchange* except when under the influence of alcohol, marijuana, and other foreign substances, you are not ready. Wait until your addiction is no longer your top priority … and union is. Find a Twelve-Step Program. There is one available for nearly every symptom of life here on Planet Separation.

A True Life Story

Once you grasp the principles it is tempting to design your own version of healing sex. Unfortunately, your instincts are programmed to retain your defenses against true intimacy. A twenty-three year-old colleague, who does a lot of meditation and yoga, was really inspired by these ideas. One day he appeared at my door, glowing. "I've just made love for four and a half hours to my friend who's visiting from Alaska for a week. It was perfect and definitely a spiritual experience. Thank you so much for letting me read your material! I did lose it at the end, but that was perfect, too."

"That's great, Rich," I said. After he left, I asked myself what Rich had read. There was certainly no commitment to a month-long approach; he had taken no time to build up an energy balance between them; and, of course, he had ejaculated. I resolved to record what unfolded.

During the rest of her brief visit his sexual control dropped off radically, and the more orgasms that occurred, the more the glow faded. Shortly after she left he stepped on a nail and hurt his foot. Then his car had a damaged tire an hour from the nearest town. (Those readers who have studied metaphysics will be familiar with the concept that our inner state controls our external experience. So an inner state of depletion manifests as draining events.)

The following week he was noticeably irritable at work, and when I asked about it, he confessed, "She's in love with me, and she might be coming back to work here. Now we'll see what kind of hole I dug for myself." I could not help noticing that he was thinking in terms of "loss" and "feeling cornered" rather than "union" and "spiritual encounter."

He cheered up significantly when she announced that she could only come back for one week the following month. Before her arrival, however, he became involved with a second woman—without mentioning to her that "Number 1" was returning. He started to question his integrity, as he was not meeting his own high standards. And when "Number 2" learned of her competition, she was only too happy to help point out his flaws. Meanwhile he incurred about $1,100 of additional, unexpected car repairs that put him in debt, something he had carefully been avoiding.

Just about the time he resolved to get serious about managing his sexual energy strictly for a higher end, "Number 1" returned in lust overdrive because of the great sex they had had before. She took personally his decision to go more slowly and was furious. When, at last, she departed, after various attempts at emotional blackmail, he said, "I really love her, but I feel relieved."

This scenario will sound familiar to anyone who has been struggling to combine loving connections with passion quests. I chose it because it shows how easy it is to become a Romance Junkie while the primitive brain rules. Even with the best intentions, you cannot lay down a new subconscious response to sexual intimacy overnight. It is not enough to grasp the beauty of the idea and run with it. You need time, structure, and a partner to recondition your neural responses to sexual intimacy. So if you are ready to try a fresh approach, use the *Exchanges* in Chapter 12. They will improve your chances of success.

Lisa's Story

Your material really hit home for me. Over the past few years I've been through two relationships with men who were close, trusted friends for at least a year before we became lovers. I was in a basement band with one of them, and the other I'd shared a secretary with before we became lovers. Both relationships "cratered" within a month or two after sex entered the picture. I remember that, right after we made love the first time, the second man said, "This was a big mistake," but he couldn't explain why he felt uneasy.

I was sorry he felt that way but figured my love for him would overcome it in due course, so I didn't push him. However, the next time we made love he unnerved me again with, "I don't always have to come, you know." This was a new one on me. I knew he loved women, and sex, so I simply couldn't believe he meant it.

I did think maybe he was worried about impotence or something, but I didn't want to rush into asking him about such a delicate matter. Anyway, I doubted we'd have that problem. Generously giving pleasure was one of my great joys and, hey, I'd heard Dr. Ruth: "Orgasm = pleasure," so "lovemaking = orgasm," right? I thought to myself, "Of course you'll come! Don't worry, I'll take care of it." And I did. Quickly, though, it felt like he was seeing me in a different light. It's hard to say why I thought so. Once he bought me a very expensive gift and I received it as a gesture of love. This clearly made him uncomfortable.

Some days later it dawned on me that perhaps the gift had been tinged with a hint of payment, as if I were a mistress or something. I felt hurt. My favors are freely given not because I undervalue them but because they are beyond anyone's means to purchase. I made sure I asked for nothing—so it would be clear our relationship wasn't a business deal. I figured that if I just kept giving (massages, meals, and so forth), things between us would shift back to the easy harmony we once had.

Instead it seemed like his uneasiness grew. Indeed, I had the impression that he would have preferred a clear "deal," because without one I registered as an enigma of whom he needed to be especially wary. Ouch! I loved this man without strings in the only ways I'd learned (i.e., emphasis on passion). But it felt like he no longer saw me accurately because of a mushrooming paranoia for which I lacked the antidote. It was painful and humiliating. And *Peace Between the Sheets* explains it all. What a relief to know there's a way around this separation problem. I no longer want to be "a great lover."

Chapter 10

In Case of Emergency

THOUGH I HOPE I HAVE MOTIVATED YOU TO GIVE THE passion pit a wide berth, this book would be incomplete if it did not offer advice on coping with a sexual hangover. Remember, there are two ways to activate the defensiveness that drives partners apart. The first is orgasm, with its subsequent slump. The second is continuous, hungry behavior that drains one partner, leaving the other agitated and frustrated. Both behaviors skew your perception of each other and lower your levels of endorphins and oxytocin. You are likely to begin wondering if you have fallen out of love.

If one of you has an orgasm, whether awake or dreaming, mark the event on a calendar. That way you can watch the timing of the hangover for yourself and learn exactly how this strange separation virus affects you. You should be clear of the worst of the distress in about two and a half weeks if you do not reactivate your Intimacy Sabotaging Device (p. 91) with reckless behavior.

The Roller Coaster

Meanwhile, fasten your seat belts because you are in for a rough ride. Here is the account of a Scottish friend:

I had very mixed feelings about trying sex without orgasm. First of all, it's not easy for me to avoid it. Multiple orgasms have always come naturally for me, though I certainly don't escape the hang-over days later. Also, I have been taught to please men even when they make unsound choices. Then, too, I didn't want to be thought peculiar for suggesting such a novel idea. Eventually, however, the chaos in my love life made me vow to give it a try. The results, while mixed, have convinced me that this is the solution. Now I just need a cooperative partner. Here's what happened:

When I met Costas, a Greek naval officer, he was charming, jovial, and full of energy. We talked for hours about The Meaning of Life, as Greeks regard themselves as the only true great philoso-phers. He also taught my friends and me Greek dancing. When we became lovers, though, we continued to go round and round. He would make love without orgasm and be thrilled with his increasing control (he said he had been a premature ejaculator before). How-ever, he never attributed his increasing sense of well-being to our unconventional lovemaking. He was sure it had to be because of some unknown factor.

So he'd renege on our agreement, ejaculate, and the trouble would start: over-sensitivity, inconsiderate behavior, and misunderstand-ings. One evening he tried to seduce a friend before my very eyes, lift-ing her off the ground, cuddling her, and asking for her phone number with me standing there. Even external events seemed to go wrong: our cars were towed or broken into, I lost my wallet twice, and so forth.

The final crash came in India where he joined me for a week while I was touring. He insisted I book the most expensive hotel in Delhi (against my advice) and he wanted to pay for it. Before he left our home city I'd asked him to promise that he wouldn't make the trip unless he would honor our agreement to avoid orgasm. He assured me—and then chose to ejaculate our first night together on the theory that "we should do it my way sometimes, and your way sometimes."

At that point I snapped and thought to myself, "Fine! You want great sex? You shall have it." I absolutely wore him out. I think we made love four times. And the following morning I demanded more.

When we got out of bed he was a zombie. He wasn't up to touring the city. After a brief effort he retreated to the hotel cocktail lounge and spent the day there drinking and complaining about how expensive the hotel was. When I returned from sightseeing he asked me to pay half of the hotel costs. Our Indian guide confessed that he had never met a more unpleasant person than Costas.

Our trip was a disaster from that point. In fact, we went our separate ways shortly thereafter, until our flight home. And, to console myself, I ran up a credit card debt it took me two years to pay off. When we arrived at the airport he wouldn't even ride into the city in the same taxi, though I had to stop at his apartment for my house keys.

Imagine my bewilderment when, only a few months later, I overheard him at a party explaining to others the benefits of ejaculation control.... Life is funny, eh?

Practical Suggestions

Intimacy builds very rapidly with this healing approach. But the downside is that a hangover of disharmony is perceived as more painful than hangovers in the good ole days when you both guarded your hearts more. Generally, by the time an accidental orgasm occurs during the *Exchanges*, your hearts are already opened, and you have come to rely on a very high level of communication and trust between you. You will miss it terribly when it temporarily fades.

When your perception of each other shifts for the worse (watch out for that second week), it feels like it is permanent. Some word or action triggers an old pattern and suddenly you are both back on the relationship roller coaster. He may look incredibly selfish and self-centered. She may look unbelievably needy and demanding, or vice versa. Both of you will see glaring personality flaws in each *other* and feel obliged to correct them, or escape. Escape leads to separation, which cuts off the opportunity to heal. Correction efforts are equally futile because true healing comes from inner strengthening and is a consequence of safe, mutual nurturing—rather than pointed advice. Wait, because your perception and your partner's behavior will change for the better as you both recover.

Meanwhile, you literally cannot feel the same ecstasy during sex because your neurochemistry has shifted. If you try, you will find yourself drawn back to conventional foreplay, fantasy, and just about anything else in an attempt to achieve the intensity of previous encounters. As that would only ensure a more painful hangover in the long run, it is better to wait until your body returns to equilibrium naturally.

The misery of dissatisfaction and confusion will pass, but *there is no quick fix.* This cannot be repeated enough. You may hurt so much for a few days that you will be certain you have to do something drastic. Don't. The only place to solve your distress is where it began, avoiding the error in the first place. And it's too late for that.

Stay Close and Quiet

 In the interim, here are a few tips that can help with damage control.

- First, sleep together every night, even if you cannot sleep, and even if every instinct in your body is telling you that you need your space. Recognize that the voice screaming in your head is just your Intimacy Sabotaging Device trying to do its job by destroying a potentially precious relationship (again) all because you obediently followed your primitive brain's prescription for a good time. Resist its commands as best you can.

- Second, promise each other that you will not make any plans about the future of your relationship until two and a half weeks after the orgasm. Trying to resolve things while your perception of each other is distorted is most unwise. No matter how objective you try to be, you are drawing false conclusions based on exaggerated impressions (born of neurochemical storms). You are sure to see things differently when the hangover has passed. If the silence between you gets too icy, you may each have to talk about your hallucinations, but try to preface your remarks with, "I know I'm going to see this differently in a few days, but...."

- Third, even though you do not feel up to it, do little things for each other without expecting anything in return, and without demonstrating your moral superiority by announcing what you have done. Unselfish service will keep some giving and appreciation energy flowing between you. By helping to open your hearts again and improve your body chemistry, this counteracts the natural post-orgasm tendency to contract, judge harshly, or behave selfishly.

🔸 Fourth, suggest that the two of you lie down and hold each other in silence as often as possible, even when it is not your turn to make a peace gesture. Imagine you are breathing in and out through your hearts.[116] This is perhaps the single most powerful healing step you can take, though the benefits may not be instantly apparent. Wait to talk things out until after an extended period of simply holding each other in silence or sleeping on it.

> *We can coexist with unpleasant feelings while taking constructive actions.* —*David K. Reynolds, author of* Constructive Living

🔸 Should a crisis come up, it may be wise to take a few hours apart from each other to regain composure.

🔸 Should anger arise, acknowledge it and release it privately, or with a specialist, as soon as possible. Your lover should not attempt to be your therapist, even if that is his or her profession. Do not tax the safety and comfort of your relationship with this potentially explosive emotion. Anger is a natural symptom of the disease of life on a planet where we have all been uncomfortably off balance with no idea how to restore wholeness, but do not overestimate anger's staying power.

🔸 It is wise to put your underwear back on and avoid intercourse for the period of the hangover. Treat your encounters strictly as healing meditations and accept that, for a while, you will not feel most of the joy in each other's arms that you have been feeling. It will return in a couple of weeks. Meanwhile, take care to avoid any passionate maneuvers. They are unconscious attempts to avoid the pain of withdrawal by substituting heat for heart.

A Man's Guide to Female English

• If she says, "I'll be ready in a minute" it means "kick off your shoes and find a good game on TV."

• "I'm not yelling!" means "Yes I'm yelling because I think it's important."

• "All we're going to buy is a soap dish" means "It goes without saying that we're stopping at the cosmetics department, the shoe department, I need to look at a few purses, those sheets would look great in the bedroom ... and, did you bring your check book?"

• "Yes" *means* "No."

• "No" *means* "No."

• "Maybe" *means* "No."

- Decide that you would rather be happy than right. That is, whenever you feel a little bit of thawing, let go of your self-righteous conclusions at least for long enough to comfort your lover. You will feel better instantly.
- Finally, though it may sound paradoxical, wait until you are feeling good before you decide if you will break up. Otherwise you may soon be kicking yourself for giving up while under the influence of a temporary desire for separation brought on by a neurochemical hangover.

Remember that as soon as you fall back into conventional sex, while coming from an unbalanced (hungry) place, you are dealing with an addictive behavior. A passion episode lights up your old neural pathways for sexual stimulation and reward-seeking. Then if you try to go back on the wagon, it feels like your best friend (the Sure Dopamine Blast) has died, and you will never feel good again if you cannot get your passion fix. At a gut level your choice seems to be addictive bliss or boredom, pointlessness, and despair. Be ready for these entirely natural symptoms. Remind yourself that they will pass in a matter of weeks. Do your best to make each other feel comfortable and loved as a dear friend no matter what happens.

> Learn from others' mistakes. . . . You may not live long enough to make them all yourself.

Be gentle with yourselves. You are trying something that is unfamiliar. Ultimately, persistence will triumph, but only if you stay together. And show some stamina because, once you derail into passion, it can be months before you stabilize the energy between you again. One passion error tends to bring about another during the two weeks following because it impairs judgment. During this rocky period the relationship may genuinely look hopeless at times. You may see temper tantrums, severe depressions, and old addictions take on new life.

The Good News

 No matter how ugly things look, miracles are possible with this approach to intimacy. Here is the tale of Isaac and Susan:

Isaac: "I want a divorce." That was how I started the conversation. I wanted a spiritual life and was ready to move on until I could find purpose and eventually some light. Susan wanted to keep the relationship together, but I couldn't have cared less. I was over it.

After three days of discussion I finally gave in and proposed a possible solution. I had just read an earlier version of *Peace Between the Sheets* and saw a stark picture of what I had been going through. I felt drained. I was irritable. I was all that the manuscript described.

We started into the *Exchanges,* me with a pretty resistant heart, and Susan with a surprising amount of love. First I ran into my fear of true love and acceptance—rather than just sexual love. Very quickly, however, we dropped our boundaries and enjoyed a different intensity. Our lovemaking has given us both a release from the material natures we had fallen into. And our perspective and consciousness widen with our commitment to this method of relating sexually. I like the excitement without the energy loss.

We were soon the only couple in our couples' therapy group making progress. I even gave the therapist a copy of this material before we stopped attending. I am deeply grateful for this work.

Susan: It seems as though all the relationships I have ever had began that downhill slide of separation shortly after the beginning. I was sick of the cycle and seriously considered celibacy as a solution. My marriage to Isaac, sadly, was no different. Fear of intimacy was driving us apart. Separation was the only solution that he saw for our deteriorating relationship. NO!—my mind screamed—not again!

That was when we came across this material. I saw how we were a classic example of nearly all the symptoms mentioned. I figured we didn't have anything to lose. So we started the *Exchanges* with some skepticism. I was soon amazed at my feelings of tenderness for this man, who only a few days before was leaving me. My heart broke open! We were daring to walk down the path towards true intimacy, and how exciting it was/is.

Every night I looked forward to the *Exchanges* with much anticipation. We actually had fun and even learned to play. . . . This was a new element in our relationship, and I loved every minute of it. We have been successfully practicing this way for months, and our lives and our relationship are on the up, up, up!

The best part about it is that lovemaking WITHOUT orgasm is so much more of a turn-on than sex WITH orgasm! This has also given us a sense of connectedness with each other and with spirit that we didn't have before. Together, I feel, we are more grounded in our spiritual practices, which is the most important thing in my life.

Author's note: Within a year they bought a house together and he soon took a rewarding new job.

Also, recognize that separation can strike your relationship in different ways during the fallout period. It does not always show up as relationship disharmony. If you manage to keep your hearts open, you will likely see your underlying stress and sense of deprivation externalized elsewhere in your life. One or both of you may become ill, face a bitter disappointment, have an accident, or be treated unfairly in some way. Difficult as it may be to accept, we are shaping our own experience of the world. The way we choose to use our sexual energy has a major impact upon our life.

A Woman's Guide to Male English

+ "I'm hungry" *means* "I'm hungry."
+ "I'm sleepy" *means* "I'm sleepy."
+ "I'm tired" *means* "I'm tired."
+ "*I love you*" means "Let's have sex now."
+ "I love you, too" *means* "Okay, I said it . . . we'd better have sex now!"
+ "Nice dress" *means* "Nice cleavage!"
+ "I like that one better" *means* "Pick any frigging dress and let's go home!"

Niki's Story

My husband and I got right into *Peace* and followed the *Exchanges* word for word. The second night he said that he never knew that he could feel so at one with another human being. That night, just my petting the back of his head with my hand as we snuggled united us. The third night he said that he didn't care if he never had another orgasm if he could feel this good all the time. I was thrilled and inspired and feeling sooooo good as well. By the eighth night I was really wet for the first time in years. I thought I'd been broken . . . but, not so. I was really turned on, and even menopause wasn't an issue; I was naturally flowing with beautiful juices and felt I was ready to have intercourse.

We were both so thrilled that we skipped the next few *Exchanges* and went right to the intercourse *Exchanges*. I was so excited to be aroused again that I couldn't think of anything else, which pulled all my energy downward. We lost the energy flow.

He has not been willing to go back to the beginning again. We've begun to fall back into old habits, and now the only thing different is that we do not have orgasms. He seems to think we have achieved something wonderful, but I know we are far from the mark. I watch myself fear that he was just willing to do anything to get me to return to our bed and now he has his comfort level, even though I know things are eroding.

In fact, it won't be long before our whole relationship tumbles again if we don't go back to the beginning and start over as if we'd never seen the book before. I'm convinced this is a wonderful pathway ... which requires focused attention on energy flow.

Chapter 11

What Are the Ecstatic Exchanges?

THE *Exchanges* ARE A RECIPE FOR CHANGING THE WAY WE make love so we can use our relationships to heal. They consist of activities couples do together, arranged in a set format. Their goal is to create a cocoon of comfort and safety for you both without any uneasiness-producing associations.

The neurochemical rewards from stillness and selflessness gradually lead to a fulfillment that is not possible to achieve while yielding to the standard sexual-arousal brain chemistry based on craving, self-gratification, and, in time, defensiveness. The *Exchanges* thus allow you to re-pattern your neural responses to intimacy while healing any subconscious uneasiness about getting closer.

The *Exchanges* were inspired by much trial and many errors and are offered in the hope that you will not have to repeat the blunders others have already made for you. So try the *Exchanges* with an open mind. You can always return to your old habits afterward if not fully satisfied.

When all else fails, try the instructions.

Structure

The *Exchanges* are divided into two Phases. The first, the Nurturing Phase, is primarily a "clothing-on" Phase. Some of the *Exchanges* in the later Healing Phase include intercourse. So if you need to discuss birth control issues or arrange for medical tests, it is time to do it. Stay in a Phase until you have completed all of its *Exchanges*.

Each *Exchange* begins with some information, followed by a *Time Out* and *Activity*. The *Exchanges* intentionally call for a gradual increase in physical intimacy. If you exceed their pace, you defeat their power to replace subconscious uneasiness with contentment. Make an effort to do one *Exchange* a day, but trust the flow of events. However, do your best to complete the first fourteen (the Nurturing Phase) in less than four weeks. Intercourse is very nourishing, so you do not want to delay it indefinitely. It is ideal if you can go away together for the seven days of the second Phase.

Think Healing, Instead of Sex

It helps to adopt a mindset of "this is not about sex; it is about healing each other." Remember, the goal is to re-pattern your subconscious. You are shifting the conventional associations between sex and craving to associations between sex and mutual feelings of giving, gratitude, ease, and peace. As explained in Chapter 3, the first set of associations is like a drug high that leads to a hangover and separation. The second is a heart high that increases your sense of well-being and desire for union.

The *Exchanges* themselves are simple, relaxed, and not especially demanding. They call for no bizarre positions or other performance challenges. They are designed to allow you to feel secure and relaxed with each other as you open to deeper intimacy. If you choose to cheat by thrusting or crawling on top of your partner when it is not advised, it is because your primitive brain is angling for an accidental crash, which will imperil the intimacy building between you. Conventional foreplay and sex are, in part, compelling because they rapidly create the emotional distance that your subconscious Intimacy Sabotaging Device finds comforting.

You are now attempting to heal the fear of intimacy behind the urge for separation. It only succumbs to regular loving contact without inflaming your cravings. As you go through the *Exchanges,* questions may come up about their effectiveness and about your relationship. Do not try to answer these or resolve your doubts. Instead, be consistent so you can evaluate the *Exchanges'* rewards objectively. The results are likely to answer most of your questions.

Approaching the *Exchanges*

There is no need to read all of the *Exchanges* before beginning, but as you go forward read each new *Exchange* out loud. They often call for discussion. They may be done at any time during the day or night. Natural lighting, such as a candle or open fire, enriches evening experiences.

The *Exchanges* call for a spirit of innocence, which flowers in complete privacy, without interruption. Ensure that children, pagers, pets, phones, and visitors will not lead to distractions. Take turns preparing the environment with gentle music, pleasant scents, extra pillows, massage oil, and non-alcoholic natural beverages.

On days when you are not ready to begin a new *Exchange,* make sure you still do a *Time Out* of your choice before falling asleep. Otherwise emotional separation can blossom and communication declines.

What if you feel like snuggling when you are not officially doing an *Exchange?* Enjoy! But stay within the limits of intimacy of the *Exchanges* you have completed safely. For example, avoid disrobing or genital contact ahead of schedule. Also resist vigorously rubbing your genitals on your partner or reaching

A Man's Guide to Female English [Further Studies]

+ If she says, "It's your decision" it actually *means* "The correct decision should be obvious by now."

+ "We need" *means* "I want."

+ "Do what you want" *means* "You'll pay for this later."

+ "You have to learn to communicate" *means* "Just agree with me."

+ "We need to talk" *means* "I need to complain."

into your partner's clothing. Feeding frenzy behavior will leave you hungrier than ever. If you focus instead on your gratitude for having your partner in your arms, and genuinely pamper one another, you will find your encounters surprisingly fulfilling.

It is also helpful to avoid rich, heavy meals, caffeine, alcohol, and other substances that alter natural feelings at least for two hours immediately before your encounters, if not entirely. Substances that alter clarity can sabotage the best of intentions. A diet that relies heavily on fresh fruit and vegetables and contains little meat and dairy may also help you experience heightened states more easily. In general, try to allow an hour or two after eating before each *Exchange*.

Most *Exchanges* take about a half hour. If you do not feel calm, clear, and ready to begin a new one, simply repeat an earlier *Time Out* and skip doing an *Exchange*.

If possible, ask another couple you think might enjoy the *Exchanges* to begin them when you do. It can be very helpful to share regular feedback with others who are trying to reorient their lovemaking. Make no effort to stay on the same schedule as your friends, however.

Intimacy builds rapidly using the *Exchanges,* but there is no need to spend every minute together. Instead why not use the energy you are creating to do something you have been putting off? Express your creativity, cheer a sick friend, do a brilliant job at work, study with intense concentration, or clean out a closet. Your increasing inspiration and efficiency may surprise you.

Make your partner the prime focus of your nurturing. You are helping each other open your hearts. It is nearly impossible to rediscover a healthy vulnerability if one of you is chatting on the phone regularly to a former lover. Whatever the future holds, let the present be a focus on genuine togetherness.

Do not masturbate before beginning the Exchanges. It is logical, but mistaken, to assume that if you release your sexual tension you will be more at ease during the *Exchanges.* Instead, try a new approach to gaining peace of mind: mutual nurturing. (See Chapter 2.)

Special Circumstances

What if you have only a few days to spend together?

Despite the gifts from intimacy, it can be surprisingly painful to start the *Exchanges* in a futureless situation, or non-relationship. They work quickly, creating a powerful desire for more closeness. When it is not forthcoming, it is distressing. So it is not advisable to use them in such circumstances.

   If you choose to start them anyway, do not skip any. Resign yourselves to the shallow end of the pool. Deep diving ahead of schedule opens you up too quickly. It will leave you acutely uncomfortable in the weeks following your imminent separation in ways you cannot foresee or prevent. You may, for example, experience dream orgasms or a severe sense of deprivation. So stick to the *Exchanges* in order. And if you find yourselves together in the future, begin again at the beginning. Let stable harmony, rather than traditional consummation, be your goal. You will both be stronger, happier, and more deeply satisfied.

What if you are in an established relationship?

You face a challenge. For the period of time you experiment with the *Exchanges,* accept that the purpose of your relationship is radically different. Whereas hunger and discharge of energy, or comfortable stagnation, may have played major roles before, determined giving and careful protection of each other's well-being now command center stage. This can be disorienting.

> If they can put a man on the moon, they ought to be able to put 'em all up there.

   To make the adjustment easily, take a moment to get back in touch with the tingly feelings you had for each other when you first met and began flirting, before you ever had sex. You might each separately write down at least three adjectives that describe how you were feeling at that time and then tell each other. Take the *Exchanges* step by step. Even if you think you are as familiar to each other as old slippers, surprises are in store.

What if you have an addiction?

See Chapter 9, the section entitled "Advice for Wilted Plants," (p. 157).

For this purpose, frequent marijuana use is an addiction because it tends to weaken willpower and promote irresponsible rationalizations for yielding to cravings.

What Worked

Although I am sure you have the key concepts down by now, I decided it would be useful to summarize what actually worked and what did not. If you learn the easy way, ignore "What Did Not." If, like me, you learn the hard way, read "What Did Not" too. It *may* shorten your learning curve.

CLEAR UNDERSTANDING. When I first became interested in sacred sex, I thought it was all about willpower. I learned, however, that it was actually about knowledge. Once I understood that I could not make any progress in learning this while still triggering my old neurochemical reward system, an ancient mystery began to reveal itself in modern, easily comprehensible terms.

Seen from this new vantage point, visual stimulation (especially for men), passionate kissing, traditional foreplay, and vigorous intercourse were not inferior. They were just especially ... fruitful. That is, over the millennia, those who engaged in them tended to produce more babies—with similar inclinations. So thanks to all the fun our ancestors had, we have lizard brains that immediately reward us for just thinking about such activities. Even worse, once stimulated, our natural response is to crave more and more, and to feel deprived if we do not dance to biology's tune.

Fortunately there are ways around this mechanism. The first is to keep your dopamine needle out of the red zone. When you feel your sexual energy rising, channel it consciously into gratitude and unselfish affection for your partner. Also, stop frequently and be still together. Feel your natural opiates light up your bodies with bliss, comfort, and satisfaction.

WILLINGNESS TO TRY SOMETHING TOTALLY UNFAMILIAR. I finally had to accept that none of my past learning or great lovemaking skills were of any use given my new goal. I knew lots about heating a partner up and asking for what I wanted, and virtually nothing about quiet forms of shared ecstasy or conscious nurturing. I felt like an electric bass player who had just been handed a harp. It was awkward, and at first I was not enthralled by the sounds it made, either. I would get frustrated, grab my bass, and get another shocking reminder that it was time to master a new skill.

Slowly I learned that touch based on giving opens the heart in profound fulfillment, and that ecstatic shared stillness does exist. Best of all, I learned that these activities can be combined with intercourse. But I did not reach this new territory until I completely abandoned the familiar and made these new activities my sole focus for an extended period of time. This type of union is totally different. It feels different. Its rewards feel different. And I had to be willing to build a completely new foundation before I could accurately judge which was most satisfying.

SLOW APPROACH. Eventually I accepted that, although I was smart enough to figure out what made conventional sex so treacherous, I was not smart enough to get around the problem without careful preparation. That is, I had to retrain myself, slowly, to a different set of neural responses when it came to intimacy. It was humbling to realize that there were no shortcuts.

I once read that ancient Tantra practitioners would spend a year or more in disciplined celibacy, preparing for a single ritual sexual encounter. That seemed an absurdly long time to me, until I realized that it had taken me even longer to select the right trajectory for genuine progress. However, I firmly believe that such a long wait is not the key, and that having a partner can make this far easier to learn once we correctly analyze the challenge.

UNWAVERING INTENTION. Force of will is of limited use on this journey. So are good but flimsy intentions. Until my intention to change over from one neural reward system to the other was total, I subconsciously remained aligned with the status quo.

Some spiritual sources speak in terms of two inner voices from which we choose to take direction. I think of those voices as the two different neural reward systems. One rewards generosity, tranquility, and closer bonding. The other rewards self-gratification and fertilization efforts. It took a while, but eventually I determined to hear only the first voice when I made love.

CONSISTENCY. When I trained my dog, consistency was more important than anything else. Otherwise he naturally assumed that commands were mere suggestions. So it proved with my brain. I was trying to lay down a new habit. And I discovered that the more consistent I was, the more rapidly I got through the uncomfortable period of hyper-vigilance, and the sooner I could relax into the rewards.

On the other hand, I got some things right from the start. My partner and I slept together loyally, even when suffering from distressing separation hangovers. And we never deliberately climaxed or tried to make each other climax.

SPIRITUAL ASPIRATIONS. This was another tough one. Years of slavery to biology's primitive reward system had left my partner with a deeply-embedded impression that he was, in fact, a lizard. He had pretty much accepted the dimensions of his terrarium, padded it with a couple of substance dependencies, and hunkered down for the duration. Uncomfortable as it was, it was home. And despite his façade of enthusiasm, he was skeptical about forsaking familiar territory in favor of "some pie-in-the-sky summit."

Fortunately I had read a lot of fairytales as a child. So I found it easy to believe the spiritual sources that insisted there was a prince inside every human reptile. I acted as a sort of annoying cuckoo clock, announcing periodically that it was time to wake up and start climbing again.

Any of the sources mentioned in Chapter 8 can furnish encouragement should you lose sight of the goal. We all have this untapped potential for synergy between partners. We misplaced the keys, but they are once again visible. So get inspired.

A Woman's Guide to Male English [Further Studies]

+ If he says, "Do you want to go to a movie?" it actually *means* "I'd eventually like to have sex with you."

+ "Can I take you out to dinner?" *means* "I'd eventually like to have sex with you."

+ "May I have this dance?" *means* "I'd eventually like to have sex with you."

+ "What's wrong?" *means* "I guess sex tonight is out of the question."

+ "You look tense. Let me give you a massage" *means* "I want to fondle you."

WILLINGNESS AND PERSISTENCE. Both partners have to share the same goal in order to make lasting progress. On the other hand, it takes time and correct cultivation of sexual energy to shed one's reptilian self-image. So be patient with any partner willing to keep trying. With all the mistakes we made, persistence turned out to be vital. My partner and I grudgingly, but willingly, set aside resentments, backed up, and slowly started again whenever we reached a *cul de sac.*

Finally we learned to hold our course and wait for the benefits to materialize. This was unnerving. After all, with conventional sex, we could push any of a number of buttons and be guaranteed a nice dopamine buzz in our brains (and not feel the hangover until later). With this new approach, though, progress was not so linear. The full advantages of openheartedness and stillness only dropped in as our nervous systems reorganized themselves. This meant spending time in a sort of void that was very unfamiliar.

What Did Not Work

ARROGANCE. I thought I could best biology using raw logic. I had figured out there was a weak point in humanity's design that biology exploited, but first I assumed that I could design my own program based on the best of both approaches to sex. I would avoid orgasm and keep all the other things I liked about sex: spontaneity, foreplay, seduction maneuvers, going for the edge, and so forth.

I was wrong. My primitive brain had been in the driver's seat for a long time, and my neural pathways had been chiseled out by its relentless urgings. Sexual arousal was like a road with deep ruts—even when I stopped before I reached biology's preferred destination. In short, passion itself was the problem. Even when I avoided orgasm, too much dopamine slowly but inexorably led to selfishness, defensiveness, inflamed (or decreased) libido, and a sense of despondency. Another dead end. Another fresh start.

PARTNER PLEASING. A friend who read an earlier draft of this book employed the suggestions for managing sexual energy while celibate with impressive success, and was blessed by a new partner only a month later. He wrote:

We made love on our second date because it just felt right. To my amazement I controlled myself with ease, but I don't think your ideas work very well for new lovers. It would have seemed awkward, or forced, to suggest such a structured approach. Maybe we'll try the ideas later. —Nicola

His relationship lasted less than three weeks. If you want to try these ideas with a partner, make sure that he or she has a chance to read this material before the two of you take your clothes off, or even engage in passionate kissing. Once the dopamine is pounding in our primitive brains, we find any suggestion not aligned with fertilization behavior highly suspect. However, the same material, calmly read with a chance to reflect on past experience, can inspire the dedication necessary for radical healing.

My standard partner-pleaser was:

I can sense we're off the track here, but maybe if I'm very generous and giving this time, he'll be equally generous next time and will wholeheartedly try this other approach with me.

Human beings, who are almost unique in having the ability to learn from the experience of others, are also remarkable for their apparent disinclination to do so.

—Douglas Adams

Wrong. I was not helping my partner learn a new habit by ensuring he received a reward (worse yet, half a reward) for moving toward his old habits. Not surprisingly, he became resentful and depressed when we had to back up. I had been reinforcing his dopamine reward system by continuing to participate on its terms. Eventually we had to go through a second, very uncomfortable period of withdrawal before we could make progress.

It is unrealistic to think we can transition to this new approach while continuing to trigger most of the usual dopamine rewards during lovemaking. Remember, our lizard brain is always there. It knows only one trick: how to reward us for things it has rewarded us for since our ancestors began playing around in matter. We can never teach it a new song. We can only teach ourselves to listen to a different channel until our new channel sounds truly heavenly.

Spiritual evolution is dependent upon inner peace, fulfillment, and openhearted connectedness with others. These qualities are associated with high levels of oxytocin and endorphins. By contrast, high levels of dopamine (and prolactin) are associated with cravings, addiction, depression, lost libido, and separation.

BENDING THE RULES. Whenever we bent the rules, it turned out we were listening to our lizard brains. Here are some sample broadcasts:

- I don't think it will cause a problem if I take my shirt off ahead of schedule.
- I can't help it, I'm a guy.
- OK, I'll try this stillness thing, but I still have to grab your butt.
- I will show you the power of the feminine with this seductive little move of my hips.

It is impossible to learn this if you are doing it for the traditional, self-serving motives that have been behind male/female relationships for so long. When we play by biology's rules, it is like entering a casino. The dealer always wins.

RESISTANCE. Biology will do everything it can to keep you in the casino so you duplicate as many genes as possible before you give up and die. Remember, we begin this journey with very dim spiritual vision. We see and feel only bodies that seem to have a limited capacity for pleasure before they decay, so it seems wise to grab as many thrills as possible in the meanwhile. Such thinking hastens our deterioration and blinds us to our potential for regeneration through union.

Here are some of the thoughts that held us back:

- I can't do this—it's too hard.
- I'm not spiritually advanced enough for this yet.
- How do you know we're not chasing a wild goose?
- I'm too tired.
- What's the rush?
- Why can't I just do it the usual way till I tire of it?
- I am who I am and I can't change that.
- Maybe I'd be better off with someone else.

These thoughts were like chains. And they had precisely the strength that we gave them. Had we yielded to them, we would soon have been too fearful of intimacy and too discouraged to keep trying.

1001 Arabian Nights contains the tale of a woman who scaled an enchanted mountain in an attempt to rescue her brothers. Before she began the climb, a convenient mystic warned her that she would hear loud, sinister voices just behind her at each step. The voices would threaten and ridicule her to cause her to turn around. But if she turned around she would instantly be transformed into a stone statue—as had her brothers.

Instead of trusting her willpower, she humbly inquired of the sage whether she could stuff her ears with cotton. He replied that she was free to try. With the cotton in her ears she could still hear the voices, but they were not overpowering enough to divert her from her goal. Resolutely, she hiked all the way up the mountain and freed her brothers from their enchantment.

The *Exchanges* are cotton. Use them.

Chapter 12

The Ecstatic Exchanges

The Nurturing Phase: Opening the Heart

 (Fourteen Exchanges)

THIS PHASE OF THE *Exchanges* CAN HELP YOU CALM AND balance your nervous systems. Are you ready? To find out, use the checklist below.

Readiness Checklist

HIM   HER

❑   ❑   I am prepared to spend the entire night, every night, with my partner while doing the *Exchanges*.

> [NOTE: If you cannot commit to this, the physical separation in your relationship will leave your old patterns unhealed. It would be best to defer sex or stick to your present way of doing things until you can make this commitment.]

_____(date) **(HIM)** My last genital orgasm (whether during dream, masturbation, or intercourse) occurred on this date

❑   or was more than two weeks ago.

_____(date) **(HER)** My last genital orgasm (whether during dream, masturbation, or intercourse) occurred on this date

❑   or was more than two weeks ago.

[NOTE: It is ideal if you can wait to begin the *Exchanges* at least two weeks after either of you has had a genital orgasm. Orgasm temporarily clouds perception and weakens desire for lasting intimacy. It also strengthens a craving for hot sex, hampering your ability to heal each other unselfishly. So especially if you are not yet living together, it would be wise to wait.

Some of us cannot get past our orgasm addiction, however, without a partner's loving energy. So if you wish to begin immediately, go ahead. Just stay within the boundaries of the *Exchanges*. Expect biology to dictate unsound instructions to you for about two weeks. Ignore them. Do not lie on top of your partner until the two weeks have passed.]

❏ ❏ I am not intimately involved with anyone other than my partner. I am willing to be monogamous while trying the *Exchanges*.

❏ ❏ I recognize that the goal of the *Exchanges* is to heal, rather than preserve, all forms of subconscious uneasiness between the sexes induced by millennia of primitive brain programming.

[NOTE: The *Exchanges* are not recommended for same-sex partners because any balance achieved is likely to be too fragile for long-term gains.]

❏ ❏ I will remain at a level of intimacy I am comfortable with and only go forward when I feel ready. I will not push my partner to go faster.

❏ ❏ If I am addicted to drugs, alcohol, or anything else I could use to keep from committing myself completely to my primary relationship, I will give it up while trying the *Exchanges*. If I backslide on the addiction I will still spend every night with my partner, but I will not do an *Exchange* while my clarity is impaired.

❏ ❏ While we are doing the *Exchanges* together, I will give generously to my lover on every level, in and out of the bedroom. I understand that unless I do, I will unintentionally drain my partner, defeating the purpose of the *Exchanges*.

❏   ❏   I understand that I can end my participation at any time, but I agree to inform my partner outside the bedroom, before I begin the next *Exchange,* if I don't want to continue.

❏   ❏   Even if I don't feel like doing a new *Exchange,* I will do a *Time Out* before falling asleep.

❏   ❏   My motive is to heal. I am not using the *Exchanges* as an excuse to seduce my partner. Yet I also understand that we may not be each other's ultimate partners, so I will let go of our physical relationship and move on without rancor if appropriate.

❏   ❏   I am willing for my relationship to be a source of comfort and healing, and I will let go of all expectations/past learning to try this new approach.

If you can check all of these, you are ready. If not, your experience of the *Exchanges* is likely to be mixed. It would be better if you did not try them.

Suggestions for the Nurturing Phase

COVER UP. As you begin the *Exchanges* there may be a temptation to combine visual stimulation with the joy of closeness. This can be true because you have been too long deprived of intimate contact, or it may happen because you are in a rut, born of past sexual habits that made visual stimulation a "rewarding" biological trigger.

The cure is simple: keep some clothing on for the Nurturing Phase of the *Exchanges* even if you have already seen each other nude. An exchange of loving energy occurs even through fabric. Let the energy surprise you. It, not your vision, is the key to feeling deeply nourished. Visual stimulation tends to leave you hungry. Gentle touch allows you to give, creating feelings of wholeness.

Men are often warmer than women. If he is in the habit of sleeping in the nude, he may remove his underwear when he is ready to fall asleep and replace it upon waking. She should keep at least a tee shirt and underwear on, however, throughout this Phase.

KEEP COOL. Hugging seems to cause little problem while some clothing is on. Forceful thrusting or simulating conventional intercourse, though, is ill advised even with clothing on. It can ignite an insatiable, grabby mentality—and trigger defensive feelings. It is impossible to stay in your heart when all you can think about is how much you want to climax. So do not intentionally heat each other up. (And do not roll around on each other until two weeks have passed after either partner's last peak orgasm.)

If you are feeling especially energetic, you can release the pressure by dancing, exercising, or stretching.

CIRCULATE ENERGY. If you feel uncomfortably aroused after or during an *Exchange,* circulate your sexual energy to regain your peace of mind. Simply close your eyes, tighten the muscles around your perineum (the area between the genitals and the anus), and imagine drawing the energy up your spine to the top of your head as you inhale. Then draw it down the front of your body and store it in your navel. A few of these deep breaths will restore your composure.

BE A GUARDIAN. Experience has shown that it is best if one partner acts as a Guardian for each *Exchange.* Otherwise, no one wants to say "whoa." If the Guardian senses the temperature rising too rapidly, he/she takes whatever measures are necessary to cool things down. Suggested techniques are:

- Vigorously scratching or rubbing your partner's scalp. This feels good and moves everyone's attention upward.
- Holding your partner in spoon and resting a hand lovingly on his penis, or her chest, until things calm down.
- Quietly saying, "Inhale" and then sitting up straight, or lying together in each other's arms, breathing deeply and slowly, and circulating your energy until you are calm and centered.
- Sitting next to your reclining partner and lightly, gently stroking his or her torso, arms, and legs, avoiding genitals.
- Cracking a joke to halt the momentum.
- Gently stroking his/her face with love.
- Looking into each other's eyes.

- Meditating or praying for inner peace.
- Touching the space over each other's heart.
- Having your partner lie, face up, in front of you as you rest your partner's head in your cradled hands without moving.

> *Extreme measures can be appropriate. The Taoist lovemaking manuals suggested keeping a bowl of ice water by the bed for him to dip his penis in. . . . So do whatever it takes!*

RELAX. Remember, your primitive brain has an agenda when you are in bed with a lover. If you want to regain control of your love life, stop striving. Let your intimacy be as unforced as breathing.

BE PATIENT. It is not unusual for the first Phase to go on for more than two weeks, so enjoy this time together as you wait for your sexual energy to stabilize.

HAVE FUN. If you have time and lots of energy, begin your *Exchange* with an *Adventure* from Appendix I.

MATERIALS. Unless otherwise noted, the only materials you will need for the *Exchanges* are pens, paper, and massage oil.

Practice Makes Perfect

The *Exchanges* are like athletic drills. They are somewhat repetitive and artificial, but they help you develop skills you will use when you make love without them. They do not guarantee that you will stay on track. However, they can steer you around the most common pitfalls. As you go through the *Exchanges* be on the lookout for activities you like well enough to add to your repertoire permanently.

Are you and your partner beginning your relationship with the *Exchanges?* If so, they can help clear any uneasiness about getting closer and launch you safely into intercourse. It is common to have a lot of PEA, a stimulating neurochemical, flowing through your system at the beginning of a relationship. It is thrilling but destabilizing, and it leaves you vulnerable to biology's insidious commands. A slow, deliberate approach can free you to experience the joys of closeness without succumbing to biology's plans for your love life.

Foul-Weather Warning

If either of you has a genital orgasm during this Phase, you should remain in this Phase for two weeks beyond the orgasm, with some clothing on, still doing a *Time Out* and, preferably, an *Activity* or *Adventure* (from Appendix II) each day. Dream orgasms count, too. Often they signal that energy is flowing backward. That is, one (or both) of you is still draining the other at an energy level. Usually the reverse flow shows up as a goal-oriented search for more physical gratification, even if you both manage to avoid orgasm while awake.

During the two weeks or so following the orgasm you can expect inexplicable mood swings, mysterious fatigue, and distancing behavior on both your parts. Tears, overreactions, icy silence, hurt feelings, a sense of victimization, exaggerated accusations, loss of courage, resurgence of old addictions, cynicism, draining physical discomforts, and flaring tempers are likely. So is a desire to "stop all this nonsense and return to good old-fashioned conventional sex." These unwelcome behaviors may be barely noticeable at first, but they worsen for about two weeks and can even surprise you with a few nasty aftershocks beyond that time.

Remember: you and your partner are just suffering from a biological hangover. Its purpose is to discourage you, separate you, and convince you that there is nothing you can do to outwit biology until your next incarnation. Be bold. The hangover will pass within a few weeks if you stay close, remain generous toward one another, and move beyond your old habits.

There is no doubt that an inadvertent genital orgasm is a major setback. For weeks afterward you tend to be out of sync with each other. If you feel an overwhelming need to give your partner an ultimatum relating to unacceptable behavior, or simply to bolt, trust that you are oversensitive and overreacting. Get quiet and be patient. Stick around. (See Chapter 10 for additional tips.)

Exchange One:
Which Way Does Your Current Flow?

There's a huge difference between your hugs and his. When you hug me I feel like you're hugging me for *me*. You want to comfort me and make me feel loved and lovable. When *he* hugs me I feel like he's hugging me for *him*. He wants to get his hands all over me because it turns *him* on.　　　—Julie

As soon as you grasp that there are two types of touching—giving and grabbing—you have the key to healing each other. Two physical touches may look the same but have totally different effects depending upon the energy flow behind the touch. Only touches with your partner's best interests at heart will lead to lasting satisfaction. Intention is far more important than what you touch or how intimate the touch is.

If you affectionately nibble your partner's ear, or stroke your partner lovingly, his or her heart will open rapidly. If you seductively lick your partner's ear, or stroke your partner's genitals with the intention of heating your partner or yourself up sexually, your primitive brain will produce excess dopamine and throw you back in an addiction cycle. This will also destabilize your partner. Stay mindful of your intentions and consciously upgrade them instead of trying to get away with a little something more than the *Exchanges* call for.

The *Exchanges* take a very slow approach to physical intimacy because most of us have not learned to distinguish clearly between generous touch and greedy touch. We are wired to fan the flames of passion, which makes us increasingly unaware and, therefore, selfish. We need time and water wings until we can stay afloat in the tempting undertow of sexual arousal. Clearly defined boundaries keep us safe while we learn to feel which way our energy is flowing in each moment and allow our conditioned responses to re-pattern. The goal is to make *giving* touch a habit, rather than to give now and then and indulge in old habits the rest of the time.

One couple found that it was easier to set a clear intention if they began by touching each other over the heart before any other touching. Loving hugs are also a good place to start. So is looking into each other's eyes, or a brief meditation while touching.

Make sure your partner is there with you, consciously responding to your love and returning it, before expanding the range of your touch. Otherwise you may find yourself fondling flesh with no one home. That can lead to a disconcerting sense of loneliness, resentment, closed hearts, sexual fantasy, and so forth. So if ever your partner is not responding, just hold him/her in stillness and wait for another occasion.

Suggested Preparation

Choose beautiful, peaceful music. *She* is the Guardian. Attire yourselves in comfortable shirts and comfortable shorts or modest underwear. Thongs or boxers that promote peeping or over-stimulated genitals defeat the purpose of covering up. If too warm, he may remove his shirt.

Time Out

- Sit comfortably, facing each other. Pretend that you have all the time in the world. Decide who will squeeze the other's hands at the end of a few moments.
- Now, let go of all other thoughts, hold hands, and look into each other's eyes for several moments and imagine you are breathing in and out through your hearts.

Activity

- Too often words create distance or superficiality, not deeper intimacy. So let silence reign. Use eyes, smiles, touches, and flowing, unseen energy to communicate instead.
- Sit next to your partner on the bed, as he/she lies next to you. Slowly stroke or gently squeeze your partner's muscles from head to toe, without intentionally stimulating him/her. Imagine that your hands are glowing with selfless, healing energy and that you can activate your partner's ability to relax and heal with your touch. Imagine your partner's body literally lighting up as you work. When you have finished, gently cradle your partner's head or feet in your hands for at least five minutes. Change roles.
- Make it a habit to touch your partner only when this energy is

streaming from your hands. That way you can be sure you are always in *give* mode.

When it is time to go to sleep

- Relax in each other's arms. Avoid tongue kissing for now and allow your energy to balance; kissing is a powerful biological trigger. Try spoon position. The person who most wants to be held should take the inside position. Whoever is on the outside can place his/her hand on the other's chest *over the clothes.* If he is feeling over-stimulated, she can hold him and rest her hand lovingly on his penis *over his clothes,* without stimulating him, as she holds him in spoon position. This is surprisingly calming and satisfying, and can help him get comfortable with loving contact even when his penis also relaxes.
- At night, if you awaken, ask your partner, with a touch, to hold you. And if asked, hold your partner despite your sleepiness. Do not feel obliged to respond with activity, but assure your partner that there is loving attention available. Hugs, after all, are an inexhaustible natural resource.

Exchange Two:
The Joy of Giving

The *Exchanges* will gradually bring your level of sexual desire into harmony with your lover's. At first, though, you may find that one of you sometimes has considerably more desire than the other. Demanding urges are the product of insufficient loving contact, while defensive, chilly responses result from being on the receiving end of desperate gobbling.

When this disharmony occurs, one partner can feel rejected while the other feels resentful. A couple of standing rules will help while you are phasing into harmony.

- First, when you are feeling needy, give. Do something genuinely helpful for your partner or someone else. Generosity literally shifts your body chemistry, healing your cravings. Your energy needs to flow outward to restore a sense of well-being. If active giving is not appropriate because your partner is resting, then hold your partner in stillness and send him/her your loving energy. Imagine how it feels to your partner to have this loving, regenerating energy flowing all through his/her body.

⤞ Second, at any time, either of you must be free to ask for a few moments of hugging or gentle stroking (at the discretion of the giver) and be sure of receiving them. Of course, the giving partner can give as much as he/she is inclined to give (within the bounds of this Phase of the *Exchanges*). Whoever is asking for affection must cheerfully soak up the giver's gift, even if it is only the few minimum hugs. If you are receiving, do not push for more. Think of ways you can express your love that would comfort and relax your partner instead of angling for what would feel best to you.

Enjoy the glow from not exhausting your desire. Because of that glow you will always welcome union. If deprivation haunts you, focus on your gratitude for having a partner. Remind yourself that you have the power to heal if you give, and if necessary, meditate, pray or simply take a few deep breaths in and out through your heart and release them slowly. Never attempt to take more, especially under the guise of making "gifts" of sexual stimulation to your partner. Manipulative behavior, or taking under the pretense of giving, drains your partner energetically. Even if you both stay loving, you cannot build up the solid core of mutual energy needed to find true satisfaction. You will grow hungrier, while your partner's appetite declines.

Above all, be patient. With consistent generosity any uneasiness will gradually lose its urgency. Your subconscious and brain chemistry will catch up with the fact that you are no longer starving for affection or being repeatedly devoured. Try these rules for a couple of weeks before making any judgments about your sexual compatibility.

Humanity is starved for affectionate touch with no strings attached. It is the strings, after all, that so often cause male and female to cut off the natural, nourishing flow of energy between them. Let yourselves rediscover that there is an endless supply of welcome, generous contact that increases the sense of well-being for you both.

Before beginning the Activity, talk about what you experienced following the previous Exchange.

- Are you having trouble sleeping together? If so, experience has shown that it is best not to give in to the urge to separate. Just enjoy your nights together and try to catch a nap at some other time. Eventually your body will adjust to your new intention to let nothing stand between you and healthy intimacy.
- Did it feel good to give even if you were sleepy? Do you feel happy? If you do, tell your partner why.

> *Whoops! Did someone have an orgasm? If so, refer to the "Foul-Weather Warning" in the introduction to this Phase.*

Suggested Preparation

Choose some beautiful, peaceful music. *He* is the Guardian. Remember, modest attire.

Time Out

Sit comfortably facing each other, with a pillow between you to support your arms. Hold your partner's left hand while you touch the area over his/her heart with your right hand. Let go of all other thoughts and close your eyes for several moments.

Activity

- Cradle your partner's head in your lap on a pillow and slowly massage his/her scalp and forehead and temples with firm but gentle, circular motions. Do not just play with your partner's hair; move the skin over the cranium. As you massage, imagine the energy around your heart increasing and expanding. Allow that energy to move through your fingers and nourish your partner.
- When you finish, hold your partner's head in stillness for at least five minutes. Change roles.

When it is time to go to sleep

- Relax in each other's arms in a comfortable position. Avoid tongue kissing for now. If you try spoon position again, whoever is on the outside can place his/her hand on the other's chest over any clothing. If he is feeling over-stimulated, she can rest her hand lovingly on his penis over his clothes as she holds him in spoon position.

⟿ Remember: the key to healing the unwelcome hunger we have all been trying to cope with is "all you can eat" of conscious, loving touch. Use your sexual desire to send your partner healing energy. Breathe through your heart.

Exchange Three:
Use 'Em And You Lose 'Em

Have you ever truly cherished someone? Perhaps a religious figure? A child? A parent? Even a pet? You probably think you are so devoted because the one you adore is especially deserving of your selfless attention. He/she is—but so is your lover.

When you look at another from a space of caring, appreciation, adoration, or desire to nurture, you see a reflection of your own open heart. That gives the object of your affection a radiance that appears to be missing from those you do not care for in this way. In short, your degree of openheartedness determines your image of others, regardless of the shape they are actually in.

Unfortunately, we reserve this generous vision for those whom we perceive as being safe to love (like a child, a pet, or a spiritual teacher). And thanks to years of alienation between the sexes (born of the fallout from conventional sex), we seldom believe that a sexual partner is totally safe to love. Instead we soon view each other through a haze of defensiveness. This causes us to undervalue our partners shortly after we begin having sex with them. Therefore we seldom maintain the degree of mutual, openhearted reverence necessary to reap the full benefits of intimacy.

It is very difficult to see our error because our body chemistry gives us clear signals that we have reason to be defensive. Yet we would be better served by emotions that open the energy field around the heart, such as caring, appreciation, devotion, and so on. As we saw in Chapter 4, we then automatically produce the feel-good neurochemicals that intensify our desire to bond deeply with another and to nurture.

Value the golden opportunity before you. Understand that your physical well-being, your ability to experience wholeness, and your spiritual vision are all at stake in each intimate encounter. Raise your sights, because when you see the inner beauty in your partner you will see your own more clearly.

Before beginning the Activity, *talk about what you experienced following the previous* Exchange.

- ✤ What does it feel like to think of your life force or sexual energy as something you give? As something you nourish another with?
- ✤ Are you able to ask for the comfort you want without insisting on your former agenda for intimate encounters? Are you able to let your partner sleep? Or are you bent on getting what you want? Are you feeling less sexually frustrated than you thought you would?
- ✤ Take a moment right now to think of something nice you could do for your partner in the next twenty-four hours. Surprise him/her.

Uh ... Did someone have an orgasm? If so, refer to the "Foul-Weather Warning" in the introduction to the first Phase.

Suggested Preparation

Find pencils and paper. Music? *She* is the Guardian. Modest attire.

Activity

- ✤ First, think of someone (or pet) in your life whom you revere(d). Take a few moments to feel the adoration you have (or had). See if you can consciously transfer those feelings onto your partner. Does your heart open or close? Notice the difference, if any, between the reverent feelings you have for the one you adore and your affection for your partner. (There is no need to share with your partner the identity of the person or pet you are thinking of, although you certainly may.)
- ✤ Now, take a few minutes to write down at least three things you appreciate about your partner that the one whom you thought of does not add to your life. Maybe it is your partner's wacky sense of humor, warm hugs, or sunny smile. Share what you have written.
- ✤ Express your gratitude to your partner for his or her gifts with a good, old-fashioned back scratching, exactly to order. Change roles.

Time Out

Enjoy a long hug (several minutes), either seated or standing. Be as still as possible. Feel your partner's loving energy, and your love for your partner. When it is time to go to sleep:

- Snuggle each other as long as you like. Avoid intentional stimulation of your partner's genitals and rubbing your genitals on your partner. If you choose to tongue kiss, imagine that your partner's lips are the lips of his or her heart. Be gentle, not arousing.
- Take frequent breaks from kissing to breathe through your hearts, smile, and relax.

Exchange Four:
Addiction

When you think of a scantily clad person of the opposite sex willingly lying next to you, does a cookie jar mentality steal over you? That is, do you suddenly have the urge to grab what cookies you can and wolf them down before this seeming window of opportunity slams shut? Whoa, baby! Your genes are talking.

When it comes to intimate encounters, most of us have developed subconscious routines geared toward the goals of conventional sex. Because the payoff is compelling (rapid or noisy climaxes for ourselves or our partner, accompanied by brain chemical buzzes that feel great, until their hangovers kick in), these routines can be as tenacious as a substance addiction.

Some routines cause us to behave so predictably that we do not even think about what we are doing. We may then mistake our robot-like behavior for spontaneity. Even when we are conscious of our behavior we may stay in our heads, carefully orchestrating each step. Such habits get in the way of mastering this new approach.

Your new goal cannot be reached by intellect, blind passion, or force of will. It is a state of mind you relax into, and it is the product of two comfortable, open hearts. The *Exchanges* can help because they are entirely inconsistent with former routines. They are built around the principles of no demands, no expectations, and no pressure to perform. Basically they are about *not* doing. This permits an entirely different body chemistry to accompany your lovemaking.

When you first experiment with an approach to intimacy that does not feed your sexual addiction, you may occasionally find that you feel disoriented, irritable, stubbornly resistant, or totally at a loss. When such feelings arise try not to identify with them by insisting that they are "your will." They are the will of your primitive brain, which is trying to coax you into duplicating your genes. Resist falling back into your addiction on the theory that you simply want to please your partner, you have sensual needs that are not being met, or you will never again feel any pleasure if you cannot produce your passion body chemicals.

Realize that, thanks to your former programming, you are just like any other addict: you want your fix, and withdrawal is a discomfort you would rather avoid. Addiction subverts our wills, causing us to cling to old habits with their predictable "rewards," whatever the cost. In this case indulging your addiction is guaranteed to set you on a downward spiral that will cheat you of intimacy's greatest gifts.

The good news is that while you are doing the *Exchanges* you have a way to ease your withdrawal: you have someone to love. If you can focus on your appreciation for your partner, and on making it safe for your partner to open to you completely, your heart will produce delicious neurochemistry and charge up its electromagnetic field. That makes possible a true sense of oneness while it heals cravings. Every step in this direction feels so good, and enables you to feel the love coming from your partner so powerfully, that you can drop your passion addiction almost painlessly.

As you learn to stay in your heart, your genitals will surprise you by aligning with your new intention; they will be ready for action without any conscious foreplay. So trust the process and resist any self-destructive impulses.

> Tip: Be especially careful of morning erections. They tend *not* to be heart-centered. If you cuddle in the morning, begin with a "Time Out" head hold or gently rub your partner over his/her heart, or sit up and meditate together.

Before beginning the Activity, *talk about the previous* Exchange.

☙ Take out the lists you made last time. Do you have anything to add that you are grateful to your partner for? Did you find that the things you valued most in your partner were related to sexual gratification or your other personal material-plane agendas? If so, recognize that you are denying yourself the most precious object your partner has for you: an open heart.

- ◆ Did you remember to do something nice as a surprise for your partner?
- ◆ Do you feel nurtured?

Check in. Did someone have an orgasm? If so, refer to the "Foul-Weather Warning" in the introduction to the first Phase.

Suggested Preparation
Music? *He is the Guardian.* Modest attire.

Time Out
Sit facing each other and take a couple of minutes to do an Energy Circulation. Close your eyes, tighten the muscles around your perineum, and then imagine drawing the energy up your spine to the top of your head as you inhale. Draw it down the front of your body, through your heart, and store it in your navel. Feel any tingles? After a few of these deep breaths, join hands for a moment and look into each other's eyes.

Activity
- ◆ Have your partner lie next to you, face down, on the bed or on a cover on the floor and relax totally by taking deep, slow breaths. Beginning at the outside of your partner's calves, use your palms to gently rock your partner's lower leg with a slow, gentle motion. Gradually move up your partner's side to his/her shoulders and down the arm. Do the other side. Have your partner roll over and repeat the process. Remember to breathe through your hearts.
- ◆ Change roles.

When it is time to go to sleep
- ◆ Thoughtfully, safely, snuggle each other for as long as you like.
- ◆ Remember, keep it simple. If you choose to kiss with open mouths, take breaks and do not use your kisses to heat your partner up. Give.

Exchange Five:
Higher Love

Are you adjusting to being "on" all the time? You may find that you long for an energy crash to bring your level of sexual arousal back to normal. Or you may feel an urge to deaden yourself with television, pulp fiction, recreational drugs, or alcohol. Remember, the goal of the *Exchanges* is to tap into higher levels of energy that will also feel normal as you grow accustomed to them. Make an effort to enjoy your higher frequency instead of undermining it. Any discomfort will pass if you actively give your surplus energy to others while you stabilize.

Remind yourself that the urge to drop your energy is not benign. It is your biological death reflex. Give life a try. Meanwhile, use energy surges to go beyond your old limitations: paint a room, discover your life's purpose, help a friend, take a walk in nature, write a book or a song, or tackle something you have been procrastinating about.

And if the energy still feels like too much, find a way to give it to your partner. Rub his feet, scratch her back, help with a chore. It will make the adjustment to your higher voltage bearable and energize your partner as well, which will pay big dividends during your more intimate moments. Even if your partner is not around, cook a favorite dish, plan an adventure for the two of you, repair or sew something. In short, befriend your sexual arousal. Use it as a signal that it is time to share your energy.

Often your newfound enthusiasm for life will seek to express itself as a passion stampede. You may feel like you have so much current flowing that you will never again feel depleted. Be ready for this biological deception. It is an urge to go over Niagara Falls in a barrel.

While you are still stabilizing, any rush will likely be followed by an uncomfortable lull. If so, relax and trust that when your energy comes up again, it will be more centered. Remember that you may also ask your partner for loving attention.

Before beginning the next Exchange, *talk about what you experienced following the previous* Exchange.

- Do you feel at ease?
- Do you feel grateful?
- If male, are you noticing that your burning desire to ejaculate is less than you expected?
- When you awaken your partner for a hug, do you attempt to grab even more than your partner is giving you?
- In the morning, do you touch each other's hearts or meditate before you move on to other types of touch?

> *Oops! Did someone have an orgasm? If so, refer to the "Foul-Weather Warning" in the introduction to the first Phase.*

Suggested Preparation
Music? *She* is the Guardian. Modest attire.

Time Out
- Lie on your backs next to each other, but in opposite directions, either on the floor or diagonally on the bed. (Your head will be near your partner's ankle and vice versa.)
- Put your hand over your partner's heart and send loving energy to him/her for several moments.

Activity
- Partner B lays his/her head in A's lap. A lovingly rubs B's head while repeating the following phrase with as many endings as he/she can come up with. B quietly enjoys the head rub.

  "I feel funny doing these *Exchanges* because...."

- Switch roles.
- Now, each of you should demonstrate a type of touching that is soothing to you but not directly sexually arousing. Practice comforting each other using this customized touch. As you go forward with the *Exchanges,* use your partner's favorite touch frequently, even without waiting for a request.

When it is time to go to sleep
- Safely snuggle each other for as long as you like.

✧ Avoid intentional stimulation of your partner's genitals and rubbing your genitals on your partner. Just indulge in reverent touch and heartfelt kisses.

Exchange Six:
Listening

Enduring, nourishing, sane harmony between the sexes is not only possible, but natural once you learn to shift your body chemistry from passion to that of deep bonding. But there appears to be no middle ground between these two chemistries. This is why you want to steer consistently for unselfishness in the bedroom. Forgiveness, too, opens the heart, creating a feeling of safety and encouraging a beneficial relaxation response at a body-chemistry level.

So in this *Exchange* do some emotional housecleaning and forgiving. Your quarry is not a spectral warrior who stabbed you in a past life. It is any guilt you may be harboring from your own misguided actions in this lifetime. Bold adventurers that you are, you have spent time on a planet where love and fear are so painfully entangled that it has been impossible to get it right until now.

Out of balance, undernourished at an energy level, and just plain cantankerous sometimes as a natural result, you have hurt others or played the martyr. And probably both. Like everyone else, you have had moments where you were less than honest, brutally sharp of tongue, uncontrollably addicted to something, compulsively over-controlling, hurtfully suspicious without cause, self-righteously resentful, or appallingly greedy or self-centered.

It is time to accept that you have had very little choice to date. And to recognize that those who hurt or offended you had equally little choice—no matter how it seemed. Why? Because they have also been feeling agitated. Even martyrs, addicts, and other victims can draw to themselves painful experiences with feelings of helplessness. Feeling deprived, we experience intense neurochemical fluctuations that seem to justify, or help attract to us, even the worst behavior. Without the comfort of wholeness we have all contributed to the general chaos.

One way to exorcise your guilt ghosts is to get them off your chest. Share them with a listener who now understands everyone's absolute innocence—your partner. Trust is a vital aspect of true intimacy. Discover that your innocence is precious to your lover. He/she would not have you suffer another pang of guilt. The past is over. The only time you can move toward inner wholeness is right now. And you can do it together.

So, bare your soul instead of your body, and release each other from the harsh sentences of the past. *Anything revealed is off limits for future discussion without the permission of the one who shares it.* Just hold each other and talk.

> *Before beginning the* Activity, *talk about what you experienced following the previous* Exchange.

- Have you noticed any shifts in the way you feel about each other since you have been doing the *Exchanges?*
- Do you feel that your partner cares deeply for you?
- Is either of you reaching in the other's underwear while snuggling? (If so, hold off on that.)
- Have you discussed whether you need to test for venereal disease? If you do need to test now is the time.
- How has your pace been? Are you likely to complete the first fourteen *Exchanges* before the suggested four-week period is up? If not, pick up the pace.

> *Whoa! Did someone have an orgasm? If so, refer to the "Foul-Weather Warning" in the introduction to the first Phase.*

Suggested Preparation
Music? *He* is the Guardian. Modest attire.

Time Out
Sit facing each other and hold hands. Close your eyes, take a deep breath, release it slowly, and see if you can locate a feeling of joy somewhere in your body. Concentrate on this joy for several minutes. Feel it expand. How would you describe it?

Activity

- Choose a position. Either:
  - Sit comfortably, facing each other and holding each other's hands, or
  - Partner B, lie down with your head on a pillow, on Partner A's lap.
- Partner A, listen to B talk, giving him/her your full attention. Express your empathy through your eyes, or through your hands on B's head. But do not react to what is being said with gestures, nods, head shaking, smiles, frowns, or other actions that evaluate your partner's remarks or delivery. Just be there. And remember to breathe through your heart.
- B, choose one of the topics from below and talk about your feelings relating to it for ten minutes. Do not ask for any feedback. Just talk. And remember to breathe through your heart.
  - Your least noble action with respect to the opposite sex. Was it infidelity, emotional blackmail, insisting on having a child over your partner's objections, abandonment, sexual aggression? (Never mind what they did to you.)
  - Anything you want/need to get off your chest (addictions, herpes, prescription antidepressants you are taking, or whatever).
- When your partner finishes, look into his/her eyes and deliver this message in your own words: "These are symptoms and wounds from years on a planet that has been governed by painful separation. There is no blame. The past is over. We can heal best by strengthening each other." Then, hold each other silently for as long as you like.
- Change roles.

Tomorrow, and thereafter, feel free to confess any other demons that pop up. Just listen without judging when your lover is talking. Comfort him/her without words. And talk about your demons, too.

When it is time to fall asleep

- Snuggle each other reverently for as long as you like.
- Remember, just reverent touch and loving kisses.

  NOTE: You will need a cassette tape or CD player and some music for the next *Exchange*.

Exchange Seven:
Musical Interlude

❧ In the past you have used your primitive brain's plan of arousal and release as a way to manage your sexual desire. In effect, you managed it by killing it temporarily with a conventional orgasm.

Now you are learning another way to manage sexual desire. Instead of a rush of the addictive neurochemical dopamine followed by a subconscious sense of deprivation, you are moving toward gentle, never-ending waves. That is, you allow your sexual energy to pull you closer to your partner and then deliberately calm yourself. You may be astonished to discover that once you are calm again you do not feel unsatisfied.

This approach is not about a struggle between you and your primitive brain. If you are feeling inner conflict, then you are heating yourselves up too much. This approach is about avoiding craving, fire, going near the edge, thrill-seeking, and hungry behavior. You consciously keep your dopamine levels out of the red zone. Excess dopamine will leave you dissatisfied, angry, depressed, or flat.

So stay affectionate, stay calm, and continue the *Exchanges* as written. The resulting body chemistry will increase your sense of wholeness and deep fulfillment. And it will lighten the energy between you. A new experience is on the way, and it blooms in an environment of conscious giving and heartfelt stillness. But it takes time to retrain your nervous system, so be patient.

This is a musical *Exchange.* While you have the music on, experiment with some new moves (as explained in the *Activity*). Many cultures on the planet still make love for hours using lazy, almost imperceptible, hip circles in mutually comfortable positions. In fact, making love by thrusting on top of a female partner was deemed so foreign by some civilizations that it was branded the "missionary position."

How did the missionaries get it so wrong? Well, thrusting is the fastest way to fertilization. So as the Church unwittingly aligned with our primitive brains by teaching that procreation was the only acceptable use of sexual attraction, much of the West acquired this emotionally alienating habit. It is not too late to discover new territory.

Before beginning the Activity, *talk about what you experienced following the previous* Exchange.

- Were you completely open and honest no matter how dirty your linen? Did you think of something later that you wish you had said? Go ahead.
- Did you find it easy not to judge your lover harshly? Do you see that there are no reliable degrees of wrongness? That is, that insane behavior of any kind is inevitable and forgivable while love and fear are confused, and humanity is innocently using its sexual energy to trigger defensiveness that distorts judgment and causes us to make errors?
- Do you feel lighter today? Do you feel cherished?

Pardon, but did someone have an orgasm? If so, refer to the "Foul-Weather Warning" in the introduction to the first Phase.

Suggested Preparation
Each of you chooses a slow, romantic song. And one of you chooses some peaceful, instrumental music. *She* is the Guardian. Modest attire for sleeping.

Activity
- Put on the first romantic song and dance in each other's arms. Just swaying back and forth to the music is fine if formal dance steps are not in your repertoire. Imagine you are merging with your partner as you dance but do not directly stimulate each other's genitals. Kissing is fine, too.
- Put on the second song. Remind your hips how to move without thrusting. Stand back to back, and keep your buttocks touching as you bend your knees slightly and circle your hips to the right a few times. Change direction. Experiment with slower circles. With smaller circles. Try it facing each other. Try holding each other's hips while you do it.
- If the Guardian advises it at any point, sit down to circulate energy together.

Time Out

Finally, put on the meditative music. Lie on your backs and place the hand nearest your lover over his or her genitals. Without moving your hand, send loving energy from your heart into your lover through your hand with each out breath. Imagine it returning through your lover's hand with each in breath until you are both completely relaxed.

When it is time to go to sleep

- Kiss and snuggle each other without firing up.
- Tonight, when you are ready to fall asleep, lie together in spoon position for a while.

Exchange Eight:
Limitless Union

One potential block to deep union between you and your partner is the subtle belief that your spiritual path is different. The experience of oneness between male and female need not conflict with any path; it is merely the rediscovery of the joint potential that lies in all of us regardless of doctrine. But you may be setting yourself up for failure when you attempt this type of union as a path to heightened awareness if you have practiced Transcendental Meditation for years, obeyed the dictates of various external authorities on *A Course in Miracles,* or followed any of countless masters teaching spiritual-sounding ego autonomy in one form or another.

Perhaps you are convinced that you (or your external authority) have found the way to God without overcoming the anger and fear between male and female. And that anything to do with sexual relationships is a sideline. At best you see it as a pastime that you hope will not detract from your real spiritual work. Maybe it is a way to manage your sexual energy so as to avoid the energy drop from masturbation. At worst, sexual union is a cause for intense guilt.

Attitudes like these can lead to carelessness, lack of focus, or self-sabotage, the blame for which will be projected onto your partner. Worse yet, when these attitudes do cause problems you will retreat into spiritual elitism to comfort yourself. "Ah, I knew all along that spiritual sexuality was a red herring," you will confidently say to yourself as you settle back into emotional separation with your preferred brand of spiritual chicken soup before you.

However, has your interpretation of your spiritual path made celibacy (without masturbation) a viable alternative for you? Has it made your relationships, however holy, a source of peace? Or has it just made it easier for you to forgive the seemingly inevitable friction and separation? Has your path led you to a sense of creative, productive giving? Or does it merely let you bliss out while you try to stay comfortable in your own isolated mental space, ideally without demanding too much from others?

If you recognize that celibacy is not working for you, that your relationships continue to show signs of emotional pain, or that you are stuck in unproductive denial or stagnation, then it may be time to give the spiritual reunion of male and female an enthusiastic try. You can always return your sole allegiance to your current approach later.

Why not use your connection with the Divine to ask whether sacred union is the Divine's will for you? If the answer is "yes," then set aside all preconceptions and sage advice to the contrary. Reach for this method of circumventing the ego with the full force of your will. The results may delight you—and your Creator.

> *Before beginning the Activity, talk about what you experienced following the previous* Exchange.

- ❧ Did you allow yourself to calm down after the romantic dancing?
- ❧ Do you feel that you are being nurtured in your relationship?
- ❧ Are you spending every night together? If not, it is best not to go forward with the *Exchanges.*
- ❧ If you have had an argument, have you tried lying together without words, in spoon position, and breathing through your heart before attempting to resolve your differences?

> *Uh-oh. Did someone have an orgasm? If so, refer to the "Foul-Weather Warning" in the introduction to the first Phase.*

Suggested Preparation
Find massage oil and a towel. Music? *He* is the Guardian. Modest attire.

Time Out

Sit facing each other, with a pillow between you on your knees to support your arms. Close your eyes, touch foreheads, and hold each other's elbows. Be still for several moments and breathe through your hearts. What do you feel?

Activity

- Partner A is the massage therapist, B the recipient. B, lie comfortably with your head face-up on a towel and pillow in A's lap, feet facing away from A's front side.
- A, before beginning, energize your hands by moving them apart and then slowly together until they are almost touching. Repeat this motion and feel the energy build up between your hands. Meanwhile, B, clench your teeth, scrunch your face toward the tip of your nose in a tight ball, and hold it for at least ten counts before relaxing completely.
- A, put a drop of massage oil on your hands. Rub B's cheeks, nose, and forehead gently up toward you and out to the side, using movements that would feel good to you. Allow your love for B to flow through your hands. B, visualize your mask melting away, revealing your true, much-loved self.
- Now, A, rub B's temples with a gentle, circular motion. Next, gently stroke around B's mouth. Make tiny circles on the muscles under B's cheekbones. Knead B's scalp and the base of B's skull. Conclude by gently but firmly pressing the top of B's skull for a count of three. Ask B what else he/she would like.
- Change roles.

When it is time to go to sleep

- Kiss and snuggle each other for as long as you like.
- Feel caring energy flowing out through your hands and arms as you touch each other.

Exchange Nine:
Rejuvenation

It is time to go even deeper emotionally. Though you probably harbor the ideal that your erotic and loving energies flow in tandem, in practice you may unwittingly separate the two. Perhaps you stay loving, but very little sexual current flows. Or perhaps you go for the stimulation only to find that the tenderness you felt in quieter moments swiftly evaporates.

Any gap between heart and genitals is merely the defensive mechanism, or Intimacy Sabotaging Device (Chapter 5) that protects you from ongoing intimacy. Why? Because immersion in each other is artificially linked in your subconscious with fear, panic, scarcity, punishment, and even death. "The wages of sin (sexual expression) *have* been death." Death of feelings of ecstasy, death from self-destructive actions, death from wasting illnesses born of broken hearts or guilt for past actions, and death of belief in an unconditionally loving Creator. In short, humankind has been pursuing fulfillment through habits that doomed us to lifeless or broken relationships, physical deterioration, and spiritual stagnation.

Intimacy without fear rejuvenates you, heightens awareness, and can ultimately shift your perception to higher ground. At a profound level you know this. It is the deeper reason you have been trying to fall in love all your life. Of course, until now, your biological programming has taken over every time you fell in love and steered you right toward uneasy separation. Or you have evaded physical intimacy, thus preventing surrender in a shared experience.

Above all, only recently have you considered whether there was a third option that would allow mutual surrender and merging in a cocoon of safety. Habit speaks with a very loud voice. It takes an independent mind to experiment with the radical approach of healing old fears through regular, intimate contact without letting your primitive brain direct the proceedings.

Play with expressing your desire for each other through your eyes and words. As you draw your sexual desire up and surround it with heart energy, it will ultimately express itself even more powerfully in truly inspired ways.

Before beginning the Activity, *talk about what you experienced following the previous* Exchange.

- How were the face massages?
- What do you like most about your time together?
- Have any happy coincidences or unexpected gifts flowed from your time together? Do you sense the Divine trying to nourish you through your relationship? If so, are you showing your gratitude by nurturing your partner?
- Is your need for "space" less than you imagined it would be?

By the way, did someone have an orgasm? If so, refer to the "Foul-Weather Warning" in the introduction to the first Phase.

Suggested Preparation
Find pencils and paper. Music? *She* is the Guardian. Modest attire.

Activity
- Play detective. Suppose it were possible to experience your ego dissolving into cosmic unity with your partner right now. Write out the following:

HOW DO I *REALLY* FEEL ABOUT MERGING?	
I'd be afraid of . . .	*The good things would be . . .*

- Any uneasy feelings go in the first column. Do not make yourself wrong for any anxiety you feel. Just get in touch with your reservations and do your best to describe them honestly.
- Any feelings of enthusiasm for closer union go in the second column. Describe exactly what you feel when you imagine merging.
- When you have both finished, examine your fears together. Accept that apprehension will remain until you learn to keep your hearts open. Yet, even now, you do not have to believe in your fears. After

all, they could merely comprise an old baseline pattern adversely affecting your ability to open your heart in the present.

↝ Write affirmations that will help you release your old programming. For example, if you feel like merging would be a dangerously emotionally intense experience, you might affirm, "An experience of merging is natural and allows me to feel more loved." Write an affirmation for each fear. When these old patterns haunt you, remind yourself of your affirmations.

↝ Next review your "good things about merging" list together. Take a moment to feel what true union would be like. Can you feel tingling? Expansion? How does the area around your heart feel?

Time Out

↝ Have your partner lie down and remain still. Sit at his/her head, with your hands on his/her shoulders. Gently rock from side to side as you alternately press on your partner's shoulders. Walk your hands down your partner's upper arms and back up to his/her neck. Then walk onto your partner's pectoral muscles (next to the shoulders), still rocking. Continue for several minutes. When your partner is thoroughly relaxed, place your hands over your partner's heart and be still for at least a minute.

↝ Change roles.

When it is time to go to sleep

↝ Practice your partner's favorite comforting (non-erotic) touch as you snuggle.

Exchange Ten:
The Heart and the Intellect

The ancient wisdom of the Chinese Taoists, the Indian Tantra practitioners, the earliest (pre-Roman) Christians (as revealed by the Gnostic Gospels), and even Plato suggest that behind the illusion of separate male and female egos there is only one cosmic being, pulsating with current. That current flows between two poles, one male and one female. The two poles are not separate. Indeed their union is so dynamic and powerful that its potential is beyond our current ability to imagine for as long as we feel separate.

Fortunately we can teach ourselves to feel that dynamic union by safely charging each other up to new levels of perception that allow us to experience our oneness. As we make it safe to love, our hearts begin to generate powerful electromagnetic fields that extend our perception beyond the physical, and synchronize easily with other open hearts. When in sync we may feel like we are uniting beyond the body. We taste union with that ultimate cosmic male/femaleness. These glimpses furnish a sense of wholeness and well-being so profound that our entire self-image shifts away from the mundane. We feel that we have entered another realm.

In fact we have just expanded into a realm that was always there and merely veiled by our self-induced defensiveness. Unfortunately, the hangover from conventional sex has kept us out of sync and left us feeling helplessly, hopelessly separate and utterly ordinary. It is apparent that we cannot change a sense of separateness to a sense of oneness by force of will. However, the wisdom of the heart is not alone sufficient to restore us to oneness. We still need our intellect to make sound choices:

- ๛ We consciously choose sexual behavior that will decrease our defensiveness. When we remove the barriers to love, union occurs naturally.
- ๛ While we heal, we choose not to separate in response to any leftover defensive emotional patterns.

As explained in earlier chapters, our subconscious has the capacity to remember emotional patterns and respond with neurochemicals that cause us to react even before our intellect has a chance to select the best response. Unfortunately, years of disharmony between the sexes have left most of us with a powerful baseline emotional response of uneasy separation in the face of ongoing intimacy. Separation feels safer even though it actually damages our health and lowers our expectations. If we act on this subconscious urge to separate, it harms our relationships.

If instead we stay close, refuse to create this artificial space for ourselves, and nurture each other, this alien urge to separate passes in a matter of days. Eventually the unmistakable benefits of this new approach to sex establish a new intimacy baseline—one that welcomes life-enhancing closeness while also allowing both partners to pursue their own interests. Union becomes a harmonious dance rather than a power struggle.

Before beginning the Activity, *talk about what you experienced following the previous* Exchange.

✤ Are you spoiling each other with thoughtful gestures and gifts? Is one of you giving more than the other? If so, the one giving less should give more so the flow is more balanced.

✤ Do you find that you are more open to other people?

✤ Do you feel more powerfully male if you are a man? More like relaxing into the role of "boat" if you are a woman (leaving the man to pilot you safely)?

✤ How is your heart feeling right now?

Ah . . . ? Did someone have an orgasm? If so, refer to the "Foul-Weather Warning" in the introduction to the first Phase.

Suggested Preparation

Find massage oil and towels. Fill the tub or a dishpan with warm, slightly soapy water. Music? *He* is the Guardian. Modest attire.

Time Out

Hold each other comfortably, sitting up if possible. As you breathe through your hearts silently visualize the electromagnetic fields around your hearts getting larger and more powerful. Feel yours pulsing. Imagine it coming into synchronization with the rhythm of your partner's heart field. Feel your heart producing the neurochemicals that help you bond deeply with each other.

Activity

✤ If possible, soak your feet together in the tub or dishpan. If not, take turns. After ten minutes, tenderly dry each other's feet thoroughly and give each foot a kiss. Exchange foot massages.

✤ The recipient's feet should ideally be at the level of your chest, with legs relaxed and comfortably supported. Now, energize your hands by clapping or rubbing them for ten seconds, and then resting them for a moment, palms up. Sense the heat or tingling in them.

- Place the feet on a towel and rub them gently with massage oil. Allow your love to flow through your hands as you massage your lover's feet silently, using your thumbs to press as deeply and firmly as you can without causing pain. Knead each bit of surface area of the sole, penetrating deep below the skin. Then give special attention to the following:
  - the pituitary stimulation point in the middle of each big toe pad.
  - the pineal stimulation point, up from the pituitary point and slightly toward the inside of the toe.
  - the sexual balancing points (the heel, the areas just below the ankle on both sides of the foot, and the Achilles tendon area, just above the heel). Use circular movements of the thumb and forefinger.

When it is time to go to sleep

- Take turns putting your hands over each other's hearts. Consciously send your partner your healing energy for specific purposes, such as to "heal his sore ankle," to "help her through her annual review at work," to "break through an old defensive pattern," or to "release an addiction."
- Kiss and snuggle each other for as long as you like.

Exchange Eleven:
Fish Food

Do you still sometimes have the sense that you are fish food spread before a hungry fish during your snuggling? If you are the fish in this situation, recognize that the more you gobble, the hungrier you will feel over the next days. This happens because you are choosing behavior that promotes the production of excess dopamine. This leads to addiction rather than peace of mind. Eventually it will push you until you reach your primitive brain's goal: genital orgasm.

You have probably repeated this pattern in the past enough to recognize it. Yet, if you are still basing your intimacy on hunger, you are probably also blaming your partner for any dissatisfaction. To you,

Dear Fish, it seems like all your problems would disappear if you only had a warmer, more cooperative partner.

You are right that you need a receptive partner. However, it is up to you to reverse the flow of energy between you, thus creating a space in which your partner will naturally open up. Think of yourself as a supplier instead of a consumer. Watch which way your energy is flowing. Avoid veiled foreplay maneuvers masquerading as gifts. Challenge yourself to bestow new forms of unselfish affection: massage your partner's hands, hug with no ulterior motive, give a head rub. Stop frequently and reorient your intentions. Try looking into your partner's eyes. Wait for your partner to touch you. Though it may be counterintuitive, the more selfless your motives, the more satisfied you will feel.

If you are the fish food, recognize that defensiveness is closing your heart at the moment. As a result, you, too, deliberately need to put your partner first. Be as warm and affectionate as possible and take the initiative so your partner unmistakably feels your love. Until the flow between you is corrected, confine yourself to non-sexual gifts of physical affection. You will know when you feel like opening up more. You may be surprised at how quickly the sparkles return to your intimacy. Meanwhile, be forgiving, and gently tell your partner if his or her behavior is fishy. Voracious gobbling is not what it appears to be. It is not proof of sexiness or even desire for union with you. It is a defense to deeper merging and will keep everyone feeling very depleted and ordinary. It pushes you apart as effectively as any cold-fish behavior.

Uneasiness has the effect of making us all feel like we have to look after Number One, and we tend to make our decisions based on what we imagine would be best for us. Sometimes that makes us grab; sometimes it makes us icy. Selfishness, though, swiftly leads to isolation, making us feel even less nourished, more needy, and more selfish. This is why the antidote to the separation virus is mutual giving.

Tips for fish

If you are feeling sexually frustrated, use the energy circulation from the introduction to this Phase to regain your composure (see "Circulate energy" on p. 189).

When you are feeling the urge to gobble up your partner in the bedroom, understand that you are in suction mode energetically. You are draining your partner no matter how much physical pleasure you may dish out. You are not a safe lover. Stop and hold your partner in stillness. Remind yourself that you want your partner always to feel safe enough to open completely in your arms. Your actions will shift as your intention changes.

Tips for fish food

Wordlessly demonstrate the kind of unselfish, affectionate lovemaking that makes you feel safe and open. Set the best possible example. Be honest. Your partner may be having trouble distinguishing between heartfelt hugs and hungry hugs, but you know. Respond to the heartfelt ones with non-erotic, openhearted affection and do not encourage a passion buildup. Respond to the hungry ones by suggesting that you hold each other in stillness until another occasion or until you genuinely feel like active snuggling again. Above all, do not assume the problem will disappear. It will not until your partner changes his/her intentions . . . and you open up completely.

BEFORE BEGINNING THE *ACTIVITY*, USE THIS QUIZ TO ASSESS WHICH ROLES YOU EACH HABITUALLY FALL INTO. Ignore the "A/P" boxes for the moment. *Only check a "HIM" or "HER" box if you both agree on who should check it.* Otherwise leave it blank.

During the *Exchanges*, which one of you has most often been:

	HIM	A/P	HER	A/P
1. Ready to get up and out of bed in the morning rather than cuddle?				
2. Crawling on top of the other, or asking your partner to crawl on top of you, despite instructions?				
3. Trying to reach in the other's clothing?				
4. Ready to stop snuggling and fall asleep?				
5. Asking for more touch?				
6. Suggesting that your activities were growing too passionate?				

Now, whoever checked boxes 2, 3, or 5 should put an "A" in the appropriate column to the right. Whoever checked 1, 4, or 6 should put a "P" to the right of the boxes checked. If you have more "A's" than "P's" in your column, you tend to be the fishy or *active* partner and your partner is usually the fish food, or *passive* partner.

Generally speaking, the active partner longs for more loving attention, and the passive partner needs to give more loving attention. For the next few *Exchanges,* switch roles. The active partner will consciously become the Receiving Partner (i.e., will take a more passive role). The more passive partner will deliberately take the active role and will be referred to as the Giving Partner. This reversal of roles should help to balance the flow of energy between you. (If you could not decide who should check all the boxes, and so ended up in a tie, the man should take the passive Receiving Partner role for the next few *Exchanges.*)

You may discover that these next *Exchanges* are your favorites. Often the partner who has been more active will find that he/she loves receiving more attention. And the partner who has been more passive realizes that he/she loves giving, as long as he/she is not feeling pushed.

After the next few *Exchanges* the man will take the giving role so she can fall into total receptivity. (She can still initiate affectionate attention, of course.) Her unguarded openness is actually the key to his gaining perfect control over the genital orgasm reflex, just as his increasing control will create a safe space in which she can open completely.

Just checking. Did someone have an orgasm? If so, refer to the "Foul-Weather Warning" in the introduction to the first Phase.

Suggested Preparation
Music? *She* is the Guardian. Modest attire.

Time Out
Sit facing each other, hold hands, and hum or tone together. Continue until you feel a powerful vibration in your forehead. Let it spread throughout your bodies. Keep it up for at least a full minute. Talk about how you feel afterward.

Activity

-❧ Certain areas of your body tend to respond to gentle touch by triggering the production of the cuddle neurochemical, oxytocin. Your ears are one area (so are breasts, lips, and noses). Give your partner a loving ear massage for several minutes. Remember to include some gentle earlobe tugging, too.

-❧ Change roles.

When it is time to go to sleep

-❧ Kiss and snuggle each other for as long as you like, trying out your new roles as Giving and Receiving Partners.

-❧ If it has been two weeks since either of you had a genital orgasm, try sleeping with your shirts off. Otherwise, she should continue to wear a shirt until two weeks are up. If shirts are off, take care not to fall back into classic foreplay. Keep all touch altruistic and loving. If at any time, now or in the future, she feels that she is being feasted upon visually, she should replace her shirt.

Exchange Twelve:
Mystery of Stillness

Have you tried touching each other over your hearts for a few moments when things start to heat up too rapidly? Have you experimented with holding each other in spoon if there is discord between you? If so, you have discovered how easy it is to restore harmony and a feeling of deep peace. You may also have discovered that powerful releases of old anxieties spontaneously occur in these periods of stillness.

Some years back therapists began to notice that people often went through intense releases during cathartic therapy but did not let go of the trauma stored in the body that underlay their distress. Instead, they sometimes became "cathartic therapy junkies," repeatedly releasing, without really healing. Some therapists believe that the intensity of such cathartic experiences can even re-traumatize the patient.

Upon researching the matter, therapists found that the single factor that most often allowed *true* healing was still, conscious presence:

a powerful intention to hold a space for another to heal. For example, while receiving still touch during energy therapies like Reiki or Polarity, clients often permanently dispel trauma stored in the body without directly addressing the traumatic event.

Many of us have subconsciously stored emotional trauma relating to sexual intimacy. Through conscious, healing stillness we can assist our partners in releasing it permanently. Quiet, loving touch is a potent secret that we need to share with all those we love.

When we simply change our state of mind in shared stillness, seemingly insoluble problems attract solutions. Hopelessly hurt feelings give way to new perspectives. Together we are healing the sense of isolation and mistrust that is the root of so much emotional distress and old trauma. We change our inner state to wholeness simply by exchanging loving energy in stillness. Our external circumstances then naturally tend to align with that shift.

Before beginning the Activity, *talk about what you experienced following the previous* Exchange.

- Were you surprised at the power of the vibration you felt from the humming? Did you feel self-conscious?
- Do you need to test for venereal disease? If so, just do it.
- Are you likely to complete the first fourteen *Exchanges* in four weeks from the time you began?
- Which were your favorite *Activities* and *Time Outs* so far?
- What was it like to be the Receiving Partner? The Giving Partner?

Yo! Did someone have an orgasm? If so, refer to the "Foul-Weather Warning" in the introduction to the first Phase.

Suggested Preparation
Find pens and paper. Music? *He* is the Guardian. Modest attire.

Activity
- Each of you draws yourself in a powerful pose. Make it simple and do not worry about artistic merit. Around the image, write the best qualities you already have, qualities that you desire, and adjectives that describe the ideal you. Examples might be: *confidence, clarity,*

courage, or *powerful, inspiring, joyful, loving,* and so on. *Hint:* Also think of some qualities you fault yourself for and add their opposites to the paper.

-⦿ Take about ten minutes. When you have finished, exchange pictures with each other. Add to your partner's picture qualities he/she is already developing that you believe reflect his/her true inner beauty. Also add any wonderful qualities he/she may have forgotten. Take care not to add qualities you wish your partner would develop. Just support him/her in the changes he/she wants to make. Compare.

Time Out

-⦿ He should lie, face up, with his head near her. She should cradle his head in her hands, with her palms resting beneath his head, and be still for about five minutes. He should just take deep breaths through his heart as she sends him loving energy through her hands.

-⦿ Change roles.

When it is time to go to sleep

-⦿ Kiss and snuggle each other for as long as you like, with the Giving Partner taking the lead.

-⦿ If shirts are now off, be especially alert to avoid classic foreplay when you wake up. Keep caring energy flowing out through your hands and avoid deliberately heating each other up. Do not roll around on each other.

NOTE: For the next *Exchange* you will need two light, comfortable blindfolds.

Exchange Thirteen:
Heightened Sensitivity

Strong, equal partners with no sense of lack most easily experience satisfying union. The kind of contact you have recently been engaging in, without deliberately heating yourselves up sexually, promotes that ideal sense of wholeness because it strengthens you both from the inside. But relationships have been based on mutual clutching and codependent weaknesses for a long time.

If you sense unequal behavior going on in your relationship, admit it. Do not let your partner's loving reinforcement back you into always being the strong father for an infantile girl, or a giant nipple for a grasping baby boy. Decline the role of policeman or governess. Or codependent cheerleader if your partner insists on clinging to an addiction. You cannot always be the strong one or the one required to prove your love to the satisfaction of your partner. And do not let your partner hook you with addictive lovemaking based on physical thrills. Such maneuvers reflect a subconscious death wish more than they reflect a healthy interest in sex. The *Exchanges* require two equal adults genuinely and generously seeking higher ends.

Be certain you are not rewarding unhealthy behavior just because it is accompanied by a heart-touching "I love you, Darling," a manipulative "You don't love me as much as I love you," or a curve ball like, "You always give yourself to me so completely" (as your partner pushes you past sound limits of behavior). Also be sure you are not tolerating selfish behavior because your beloved says things like, "You're an angel in my life," "I told you, you should be stricter with me," or "I'd like to give you more, but you always do all the giving." Nonsense. There are always creative ways to give. And if giving does not go both ways, it is draining.

Take care not to force your partner to choose between refusing to meet your imagined needs and yielding to dangerous behavior. This is a no-win situation. Your partner could never meet a need driven by your inner hunger. If you have been doing the *Exchanges* as written, without trying to heat yourselves up, you should no longer feel like a bottomless pit of needs. You are strong enough to extinguish destructive behavior patterns for good.

Before beginning the Activity, *talk about what you experienced following the previous* Exchange.

⚬ Are you reaching in each other's clothes? Or behaving like a hungry fish? If so, lie still in each other's arms as often as possible until you feel the heart energy flowing.

⚬ Have there been any positive changes in your lives since you began the *Exchanges*? Have any of them come through your partner?

❧ Have you thought of any qualities you want to add to your pictures? Any time you catch yourself making yourself wrong for something, just get out the picture and add the opposite quality to it. Allow yourself to create a new self-image that reflects where you want to go. Your past is past.

> *Ahem. Did someone have an orgasm? If so, refer to the "Foul-Weather Warning" in the introduction to the first Phase.*

Suggested Preparation

Find two light, comfortable blindfolds. Music? *She* is the Guardian. Modest attire.

Time Out

❧ Hold each other for several minutes, lying down.

❧ Imagine a cocoon of loving energy around the two of you, expanding from your hearts.

Activity

❧ Have you discussed birth control? Condoms have a down side. They encourage careless lovemaking when arousal levels are high. They also decrease the nourishing flow of intimacy between you, which fuels an unhealthy search for more vigorous stimulation. If awaiting AIDS test results or coping with herpes, do what you need to do, but if neither is an issue for you, consider avoiding condoms during the next Phase. If he can be trusted to withdraw in time in the event of an inadvertent ejaculation, then her regular use of a spermicide may be enough protection against any sperm that find their way into his pre-ejaculate. Take some time to discuss the options with each other and reach a satisfactory solution. Decide now who will buy or supply what is needed.

❧ After reading the rest of this *Exchange,* gently blindfold each other and then remove your lover's clothing, except for underwear. Touch each other with the goal of communicating how much you cherish your partner. Send loving, sexual energy from your heart through your hands. Feel your partner's love and warmth flowing back to you. Try keeping your blindfolds on while you snuggle. If it has not been at least two weeks since someone's last orgasm, she should put her tee shirt back on before you remove your blindfolds, and continue to sleep in it.

When it is time to go to sleep

❧ Kiss and snuggle each other for as long as you like with the Giving Partner taking the lead. Avoid heating each other up sexually or stimulating each other's genitals.

❧ If shirts are off, take extra care not to fall back into classic foreplay. Keep all touch gentle and healing or simply hold each other in stillness.

Exchange Fourteen:
Progress

Has any uneasiness come up for either of you? Releasing a lifelong fear of intimacy is not a linear process. It is more like an upward spiral tilting to the side. You feel as if you are slipping backward frequently, though overall, progress is unmistakable. Often particularly moving experiences, such as seeing a loving vulnerability in your lover's eyes, or feeling tears of gratitude for him/her well up, will later trigger profound uneasiness. And you will be sure to assign the uneasiness to some other cause. None of us likes to believe we have been tricked (by our primitive brains) into fearing healthy intimacy.

If you rock between emotional bonding and emotional distance during the *Exchanges,* stay optimistic. This is natural. Uneasiness often shows up in women as a fear they are being used, and in men as a fear that impossible or mutually inconsistent demands are being placed on them. Walk past such panicky feelings, and resist the urge to separate or even judge each other. Return to each other's arms for the daily *Exchange* with as much tenderness as you can muster, regardless of what has been going on between you. Eventually you will be rewarded with a new level of trust and safety as fears gradually dissolve. Think of it as charging up a joint battery. Inner harmony will make it easier to resolve any external obstructions to your relationship.

This is a therapeutic massage *Exchange.* If it has been at least two weeks since your last orgasm, shirts can come off for good, but keep your focus on giving. That is, when it is your turn to be the therapist, give your full attention to relaxing your partner's back, head, and neck muscles, not to turning yourself on. The healing energy you are cultivating is not dependent on calculated physical stimulation. It is the natural result of proximity to a loving, enthusiastic partner.

Before beginning the Activity, *talk about what you experienced following the previous* Exchange.

- Was affection different blindfolded? How? Did you feel more? Was it fun to take off each other's clothing without vision?
- Be honest: are you calmer than you ever thought you would be after at least two weeks of no orgasm and lots of loving contact with the opposite sex?
- Does your intimate time together feel like inhaling and exhaling, that is, like arousal followed by easy relaxation? If not, you are resisting a natural flow in your lovemaking that would serve you well when it is time for intercourse. Learn to take pleasure in both the energy when it flows and the affectionate snuggling. This way you can nourish each other for as long as you like and enjoy every moment of it.

Well? Did someone have an orgasm? If so, refer to the "Foul-Weather Warning" in the introduction to the first Phase.

Suggested Preparation

Find massage oil. Music? *He* is the Guardian. Comfortable shirts (except during your massage) and modest underwear.

Time Out

- Sit on the floor or bed, back to back. Close your eyes and breathe deeply and slowly. Inhale and exhale through your hearts.
- When he is ready, he should quietly say, "Up." Imagine a glowing ball of light at the base of your spines. As you breathe in, draw it, breath by breath, up your spines to the crowns of your heads.
- When she feels it is there and you have paused for a couple of moments, she can end the exercise.

Activity

- The partner with the most massage experience should give the first massage. Whoever is receiving the first massage lies prone on the pad or table.
- If working on the floor, and it is feasible to do so, sit astride your lover's back. Take a few deep breaths together while the therapist allows loving energy to charge up his or her hands. Using some massage oil, massage him/her in whatever way you would like to be massaged. Your lover can give you feedback with sighs and moans to let you know what is most satisfying. But do not chat. Lean forward and use the weight of your body to press harder, but avoid pressure on the spine itself. End with a massage of the head and some kisses on the neck.
- Key concepts for good technique are:
  - Slowly and strongly, *or* feathery, but not in between.
  - Stay conscious of what you are doing and how it would feel.
  - Switch roles. Or plan to repeat this *Exchange* next time so you can switch roles.

When it is time to go to sleep

Spend some time kissing each other reverently, with the Giving Partner taking the lead.

The Healing Phase: Return to Innocence
 (Seven Exchanges)

IF YOU HAVE COMPLETED THE NURTURING PHASE ACCORDING
to the recipe, your subconscious uneasiness about getting closer is
slumbering peacefully. Do not let it lull you into a false sense of security. Your Intimacy Sabotaging Device (Chapter 5) is still there, just
waiting for you to heat yourself up sexually so it can save you from
ongoing intimacy. The best defense is to lay down a new, comforting
pattern around the experience of intercourse itself and then repeat it
until it becomes more familiar than the dopamine-rush-from-passion
habit. (See Chapter 3 on the addictiveness of conventional sex.)

Planning Ahead

The easiest way to establish a new pattern is to plan your
encounters consciously. It is unfortunate, but spontaneous
sex is risky sex. It invites your primitive brain to take over. Happily,
planned encounters offer some surprising rewards. When you plan in
advance to make love there is a pleasant, but temperate, sense of anticipation. It also makes the encounter a special celebration, like a Thanks-
giving dinner.

Too often lovers snack whenever hungry where sex is concerned.
This can not only make experiences more ordinary, but is also likely

to leave you in a state of constant craving. After all, without a schedule, you do not know for sure when you will be fed next, so one of you (at least) will feel obliged to initiate sexual activity constantly. As the saying goes, you cannot make sales if you do not make calls—and biology wants you to make sales.

This hungry mindset is not harmless. It leaves the most eager partner dissatisfied much of the time, while the other partner feels increasingly drained. Both of you will likely blame the other for any anxiety. It is better to take command of your primitive programming by choosing ahead of time when you will make love. When you know, with certainty, that you will have a feast of lovemaking on a set occasion, you can more calmly turn your attention to other aspects of your life in the interim.

Planning also serves as a reminder that the encounter is part of a larger effort to master another way of making love. Such a mindset makes you more conscientious and prevents slips. A predetermined intercourse schedule also makes the occasions when you only snuggle more delicious. There is no biological goal in sight, so you relax more. It is easy to stay in your heart and enjoy the warm companionship of your partner. You may find that you truly enjoy these regular returns to the previous Phase and marvel at how intercourse is not, after all, the only point of intimacy.

So how often should you make love (after completing the *Exchanges*)? The answer is different for each couple. Suggestions:

- ❧ Skip at least an entire day between the days on which you make love.
- ❧ Make love only once per day. (Feel free to have intercourse as many times as you like during a lovemaking session, but once it ends, wait until the next scheduled occasion.)
- ❧ If you do not have intercourse on a scheduled occasion, avoid it the next day as well. This gives your nervous system a chance to calm down completely and come back under your conscious control for at least a day before you "rev up" again. If you do not take this extra day off, you run the risk of staying overheated for days at a time if events keep delaying your lovemaking. Constant desire will erode your equilibrium.
- ❧ If you have been apart for days, delay intercourse at least until

your second day together. By then you will be coming from a less hungry, more balanced place.

⚬ If you decide to be spontaneous now and then, wait your usual interval before your next occasion.

The precise schedule you choose does not matter—as long as you have agreed on one. Some couples schedule their lovemaking dates around the woman's fertility cycle. Others use astrological benchmarks. This Phase of the *Exchanges* is designed around an "every third day" schedule and begins with a slow approach. Try it for this week. It may help you determine your ideal schedule.

The Healing Phase is quite different from the Nurturing Phase in one respect: these last seven *Exchanges* are intended to be done *one per day*. In fact, if you miss a day, begin this Phase again. The more times you begin, the better. Practice will help you lay down a new habit that you may wish to make life-long. Just repeat your favorite *Time Outs* and substitute *Adventures* from the end of the book for the *Activities* you have already done. Of course, it is ideal if you can go away together for the next eight days.

There is a temptation to relax your intention to complete the *Exchanges* as soon as you and your partner have intercourse the first time. However, you will not see the benefits of experimenting with a scheduled approach unless you complete the full week.

Are You Ready?

Has it been at least two weeks since either of you last had a genital orgasm or dream orgasm? If not, return to the Nurturing Phase until the two weeks are up. Patiently allow your energy to balance. Do *Time Outs* and substitute *Adventures* from Appendix II for *Activities*. And if you have been taking a break from the *Exchanges*, with no conscious effort to snuggle each other selflessly at least once a day, you need to stabilize the flow of energy between you before proceeding. Drop back into the last Phase for as many days as you have skipped (up to a week), again substituting *Adventures* from Appendix II for *Activities*, if you like.

Now, take a moment to discuss the following:

~ What safe sex or birth control methods have you decided to employ if you need them?

~ Have you tested for venereal disease if you need to? If not, you are not ready for this Phase.

~ Do you both feel enthusiastic about proceeding? If either of you has any hesitation, remain in the Nurturing Phase until you feel ready. If it has been longer than four weeks and you do not feel ready, you may also wish to consult the *Impasse Checklist* in Appendix I.

The Heart Orgasm

If you are willing to move away from heating yourselves up sexually, the Healing Phase will allow you to raise each other's spirits consistently. This leads to a feeling of safety and joyful aliveness you can depend upon. It will not feed your passion addiction, but it will feed you. And, over the long term, you will tend to make love more frequently than most couples.

A steady diet of generous, deeply emotional affection is more nourishing than bursts of sexual hunger followed by emotional distance. My fiancé described his initial experience of this emotional depth as a heart orgasm. If you stick to the *Exchanges* you are very likely to experience this heart orgasm for yourself. It is the only way you can wrest your peace of mind from biology's grip on your genitals. Repressing sexual desire will not work over the long haul. Channeling it through the heart will. So make love to each other only as you would want someone to make love to a family member you love.

It is possible to experience the heart orgasm in passionate non-relationships, too, as any Romance Junkie will tell you. Paradoxically, however, in a non-relationship a heart orgasm will engender subsequent fear. This is because a profound emotional tie to a passionate partner triggers a separation reflex. Our subconscious will eventually try to save us from continual risky passion, no matter how heartfelt, and cracks in the relationship inevitably follow.

To move toward this heart orgasm in an ongoing relationship, consciously build up each other's inner strength and sense of balanced well-being. With a solid energy foundation you have no breeding ground for fear and you will choose to stay close and continue to nourish each other. Inner strength allows you to enjoy nurturing each other without feeling deprived, depleted, or depressed. This is the only way you can beat the "passion/panic" flaw in your design. If you do not get around it, excess dopamine will set off a sense of deprivation. No amount of love, sexual attraction, awareness, or determination will prevent you from sliding down biology's slippery slope. And indulgence will eventually cause you to pull away from your partner through anger, addiction, accident, or otherwise. Or you might push

HEART ORGASM	"HOT" ORGASM
Before...	*Before...*
• Mutual desire to make partner feel safe and loved • Calm, relaxed, caring • Lots of cuddle hormone (oxytocin) flowing through your system • Sense that you are both on holy ground	• Rapid movement • Tension • Hunger for more intense physical stimulation • Lots of addiction hormone (dopamine) flowing through your system • Mutual selfishness
During...	*During...*
• Intense feelings of love and bliss that go on and on • A sense of merging, or perfect alignment with each other • Thrilling sense of wonder, timelessness • No need for release, effortless • A feeling that this is all natural and that you have been here before and had just forgotten how	• Sense that something (biology) has taken control of you • Urgent need for release • Explosive sensations that leave little attention for partner • Emphasis on performance and quantity • Focus on the physical, rather than deeper feelings • Often hunger for more
After...	*After...*
• A feeling of profound balance and nourishment that lasts • Feeling that you continue to make love even out of bed	• A feeling of, is that all there is? • Emotional distance, need for recovery, or irritability • Extreme neediness, jealousy, etc.

your partner away with illness, clinging, frigidity, impotence, jealousy, or unreasonable demands. The separation may take a while, but it will surface.

Remember, passion feels so good because biology wants to ensure that you procreate with reckless abandon. Regardless of the initial neurochemical thrills of this course of action, a part of you definitely does not like to slide into this vortex. Each of us has an innate desire to rediscover our full potential and free ourselves from primitive brain programming. Heed this longing whenever your genitals propose that you would feel more alive if you engaged in reckless, hunger-based sex.

(Another) Foul-Weather Warning

If either of you has a genital orgasm during this Phase, put your underwear on and drop back to the Nurturing Phase for a couple of weeks. During those two weeks you can expect mysterious mood swings and unpalatable behavior on both your parts. You or your partner could feel utterly dejected. A craving for passion-driven sex is likely to skyrocket on the part of one, or both, of you.

Friction may be barely noticeable at first but tends to worsen for at least two weeks. Then it will begin to fade rapidly. Meanwhile, though, one partner or the other is likely to imagine that he/she cannot possibly go forward and issue an ultimatum of departure or escape into a former addiction. If this should happen, re-read Chapter 10. Realize that you have been tricked by a mindless biological separation mechanism. Resolve to stay together every night for two more weeks at least. Hold each other before going to sleep, even if you do not talk. Unless there is sex based on genital gratification, or one of you moves out, you will soon be laughing about any ultimatums and finding the strength to drop your addictions again.

Be forewarned. Even if you believe you survived conventional sex in the past relatively unscathed, you are playing on a different field now. Intercourse with an open heart is a beautiful event. The defensive shield over your heart begins to dissolve. Under such circumstances intense closeness itself can trigger your separation reflex during the days following orgasm. This occurs because you have inadvertently reactivated your subconscious fear of ongoing intimacy, and your inner balance is temporarily inadequate to allow you to disregard the misguided alarm signals.

Also, a partner's post-orgasm mood swings and distancing behaviors, though temporary, can do unimaginable damage while you, too, are suffering from a sense of deprivation. It requires a massive effort keep your heart open in the face of gale-force emotions of anger, blame, stampeding self-indulgence, mind-boggling selfishness, unexpected emotional withdrawals (right at the time you most need reassurance ...), sulking, and so forth. You will long to snap shut like a turtle and not make yourself vulnerable again. Or you will condemn your partner or yourself for your rotten behavior. Avoid this challenge.

And should you inadvertently put yourself to the test, recognize that you and your partner are just suffering from a natural, neurochemically-based hangover designed to promote fertilization, ensure your separation, and ultimately speed your deaths. It is amazingly effective. So it is better to wait out this awkward two-week period before moving back into the emotional depths that accompany intercourse. Otherwise you may destroy your relationship for good.

When separation erupts, admit it. Sometimes inner stress first appears in the form of illness or unexpected events that pull you apart, rather than emotional distance. Just notice that separation is separation and it puts stress on your relationship.

Tips

Monitor your state of mind day-by-day. Regardless of what an *Exchange* in the Healing Phase proposes, only continue into intercourse if you are both adequately aroused from gentle kissing and touching without deliberate, physical stimulation, sexual fantasy, or sexual stimulants. His erection need not be strong, but she must be lubricating thoroughly, without benefit of saliva or artificial lubricant.

◦ If you go through the motions of having intercourse when you are not ready, you will move away from your goal. By forcing things, you will subconsciously link intimacy with feelings of uneasiness. So only make love if you sense the experience will take you deeper. If either of you is not ready on some occasion, just hold each other and begin this Phase again on the next occasion. Allow your genitals and heart time to reconnect at their own pace.

◦ You are seeking to replace the ingrained habit of heating up and thrusting to a rapid conclusion. It will not yield without a sustained non-effort over a period of time. Avoid vigorous thrusting during intercourse and emphasize gentle movements and periods of stillness in which you consciously focus on delicious feelings of well-being. Though the *Exchanges* approach intercourse very slowly, the ultimate target is this*: when you are adequately aroused, connect genitals and ignore the urge to escalate. When arousal fades, let it go without striving to stay aroused. Connect again when you are aroused again. It is that simple.* You will feel more satisfaction in the long run if you avoid deep thrusting. When you move while connected, move slowly.

◦ This Phase of the *Exchanges* will let you discover that fulfillment is possible without performance. True satisfaction is based on inner equilibrium, not friction. This approach may be the most serene way you have ever learned something. It is a study in not doing. The emphasis is on comfort, companionship, and relaxation. It obviously bears little relation to conventional sex because it is a path to a totally different destination. You allow your lovemaking to fall into easy waves instead of trying to force anything.

◦ It is perfectly normal (and actually a good sign) if your sex drive temporarily goes into a mysterious decline at some point during the *Exchanges*. This means that the emotional split between your heart and genitals is rewiring itself. Relax and wait with confidence. Put your attention on making your partner feel safe and loved while you begin this Phase (or even the Nurturing Phase) again. Your libido will return. Allow your native longing for wholeness, i.e., sexual desire, to burn through any remaining subconscious uneasiness about intimacy.

The older you are, the more unnerving this temporary decline may be. Understand that it does not happen because your innate sex drive has radically decreased. It happens because your fear of ongoing intimacy has (naturally) increased with each past episode of relationship trauma. As you begin to open up emotionally, your subconscious passes through a period of confusion; it is not sure it wants to risk closeness again. Give your old defenses time to dissolve and your sexual desire will be stronger and saner than ever without the stranglehold of your subconscious guardian against ongoing intimacy.

- Men, you face an added challenge. You are now the pilot, while she is the boat (see Chapter 9). However, in addition to a blind instinct to use her body to stimulate yourself, you may have a habit of turning on by using her as eye candy. When you look at her do you feel a wave of reverence and intense gratitude? Or is your limbic brain saying, "Man, I'd like to get my hands and tongue and penis all over *that!*"? If it is the latter, you are coming from hunger, and you will unintentionally drain your partner's energy, gradually creating defensiveness. Women, too, can suffer from this primitive programming; so they also want to take care not to relegate partners to the role of sexual stimulation devices.

- If you feel uncomfortably aroused after or during an *Exchange,* circulate your energy to regain your peace of mind. Simply close your eyes, tighten the muscles around your perineum, and draw the energy up your spine to the top of your head as you inhale. Then imagine storing it in your navel. A few of these deep breaths will restore your composure.

- Finally, forget everything you ever knew about sex. If you keep thinking in terms of conventional sex, you will overshoot the entrance ramp to this mystery and not find it. Treat intercourse during this Phase as a mutual healing rather than as a sexual encounter. If you are ready, here goes....

Exchange Fifteen:
Not Yet

 How is your state of mind? By this
point in the *Exchanges,* do you:

	HIM		HER	
	Yes	No	Yes	No
1. Enjoy doing little things for your partner and making loving gifts?				
2. Spontaneously feel a desire to touch and love all of your partner—especially the non-genital places you know he/she loves best?				
3. Feel adored and at ease when you end a snuggle?				
4. Feel increasingly comfortable with, and loving toward, your partner?				
5. Keep climbing on top of your partner because it turns you on?				
6. Tend to focus on the activities that reward you with greater genital stimulation?				
7. Feel like you are just engaging in pointless activities until you can have intercourse?				
8. Find yourself using classic foreplay maneuvers to excite your partner?				
9. Feel out of sync in bed, misreading signals, moving the wrong way, as if you spoke different languages?				
10. Find that erotic images of other partners or fantasy partners distract you during *Exchanges* or at other times?				
11. Experience feelings of resentment toward your partner and an increasing urge to distance yourself?				
12. Feel inadequately aroused to welcome genital connection?				

The *Key* is located on the next page. Check it now.

Key

If both of you answered "yes" to the first four and "no" to the last eight questions, you are ready for this Phase.

If either of you answered "no" to any of the first four, or "yes" to any of the last four, you both need to spend more time in the Nurturing Phase. Your Intimacy Sabotaging Device's clammy presence is still spooking you with its defensive search for separation. It will vanish if you rededicate yourself to quiet energy exchanges at the Nurturing Phase level and make adoring your partner your only priority. Be patient and give yourselves time. When you can honestly answer the first four questions "yes" and the last eight "no," you are ready for this Phase.

What if you are in between these two extremes? If either of you answered "yes" to the first four, "no" to the last four, *but "yes" to any of the second four questions,* you should give serious thought to remaining in the previous Phase for a while. You are sometimes making love unconsciously, which will block progress and can lead to regret. If you decide to proceed, and your genitals consistently welcome genital connection, do so with caution. Be very conservative. Stay strictly within the bounds of the Healing Phase *Exchanges,* and ask your partner to stop you if either of you begins to stray. Be extra loving toward your partner, especially outside the bedroom. And when you get that urge to gobble your partner, remind yourself that more than anything else you actually want your partner to feel safe in your arms so he/she can open up to you completely on every level.

A goal of the *Exchanges* is to establish a perfect inner energy balance between you so your mutual magnetism sets up a powerful flow of energy. If you begin intercourse while you are still coming from a sense of hunger or defensiveness, sex will not satisfy. The *Exchanges* can guide you through the physical steps that promote this healing experience, but all true progress toward reunion of the sexes is a function of opening your hearts, and progress is not linear. So, *if ever you are not ready, do not have intercourse.*

> *Before beginning the* Activity, *talk about what you experienced following the previous* Exchange.

☛ Did you fall back into standard foreplay during the massages? If so, you are off course. Return your focus to considerate attention for your partner instead of arousing yourself directly or indirectly.

Attempts to heat up yourself or your partner set up the wrong energy flow. Your partner is dangerously likely to respond in kind. If things are heating up too much she may keep her shirt on during the next few *Exchanges* until it is time to go to sleep.

↝ Have you been using your partner's favorite comforting touch during your time together?

> *Say, did someone have an orgasm? If so, refer to the "Foul Weather Warning" in the introduction to this Phase.*

Suggested Preparation

Music? *She* is the Guardian. Use your discretion about attire from here on.

Time Out

↝ Lie in each other's arms in a comfortable position. Be still for several minutes while you search throughout your body for a feeling of profound well-being.

↝ Describe it to your partner.

Activity

↝ Take turns guiding each other into new positions using only light touch without words. Then, together, choose hand signals for the following:

- ✦ asking your partner to stop moving immediately and inhale to relax (this can prevent mistakes and also be used to savor the stillness together when you are in a heart space).

- ✦ asking your partner to hold you in a comfortable position (useful in the middle of the night when you do not feel like talking)

- ✦ telling your partner wordlessly how glad you are that he/she is in your life (always useful)

When it is time to go to sleep

↝ Kiss and snuggle as much as you like, breathing through your hearts.

↝ When you are both adequately relaxed, or if it is evening and you are ready to fall asleep move into "Prayer for Union" (see "scissors position"). Remove your clothing and lie together in scissors position, forming an "X" on the bed, legs intertwined. He is on his side, and she is on her back.

- It is fine if you are not aroused. If you are, just enjoy it. If you are uncomfortably aroused, do the energy circulation from the second to last Tip on p. 137 until you return to a resting state, and be a bit less enthusiastic in future *Exchanges*.

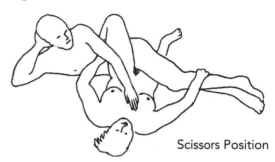

Scissors Position

- Merely press your genitals together, without intercourse, as you lie in scissors position. Circulate the sexual energy between you by visualizing it flowing into her genitals and out of her heart into his and down to his genitals. For at least fifteen minutes try not to change positions or move except to get more comfortable. When you finish, fall asleep or get dressed and get on with your day. Do not heat yourselves with classic foreplay.

- If you awaken in the night uncomfortably aroused, move back into "Prayer for Union" with your lover. It will nourish you while permitting you to relax deeply.

- If ever you suffer from pain in the genitals, you are engaging in too much physical stimulation. The pain is harmless and will go away, usually within twenty-four hours, though it can last longer. You do not need to have an orgasm to help it pass. Wait patiently and accept that you have been given a clear signal that you have been gobbling instead of nourishing each other. Meanwhile avoid stimulating each other's genitals directly.

Exchange Sixteen:
Taking It Easy

This *Exchange* includes intercourse. But it will be nothing like you remembered. It will be part of the "Prayer for Union," in one of the still positions pictured below and in the previous *Exchange*.

The key for this *Exchange* is to avoid excess hunger by converting it to gratitude or thoughtful attention. Cravings would reverse the energy flow between you and leave you feeling empty or resentful after your encounter. So, take lots of breaks and breathe together. Unless you are in a heart space of reverence, lying on your partner can trigger your primitive brain to do biology's dance, so for now, avoid lying on top of your partner when underwear is off.

Watch your thoughts to assess your state of mind. If you find yourself saying or thinking phrases like, "I just want to swallow you whole," you are draining your partner at an energetic level and need to refocus. If you find yourself saying or thinking, "I am just so grateful to have you in my life," and "what can I do to help you feel loved?" you are right on course.

It cannot be repeated too often that pushing yourself or your partner to have intercourse when your bodies are not signaling their obvious enthusiasm would be an error. If your genitals are not ready, you are not ready . . . no matter how ready you were yesterday. If either of you is not ready, just begin this Phase again, keeping the *Time Outs* and substituting new *Activities* or *Adventures* from Appendix II. You will be ready soon.

During this Phase, *be sure to admit it if there is an inadvertent peak orgasm* or even the beginning of one. (Ask each other now.) Otherwise you will be completely bewildered by the subsequent disharmony or lack of affection you encounter. Experience has revealed that the aftershocks from a wet dream (common if there has been too much emphasis on physical gratification) or from a "Gee, I Might Have" orgasm produce uneasiness as surely as fallout from an orgasm that registers 8.8 on the Richter scale. So it is better to admit any possible slip and start the first Phase again than to rationalize rolling onward. If you have to back up, make each other feel good about the delay. Trust your bodies' signals that the balance between you has not yet stabilized.

> Before beginning the Activity, *talk about what you experienced following the previous* Exchange.

- ❧ Did your "Prayer for Union" feel like a sacred act? Why? Why not?
- ❧ Could you sense the conscious flow of energy between you? Or did you just fall asleep in protest because you could not rub all over your partner? (Or did you rub all over your partner??) For this *Exchange* focus on those subtle energy flows. They may surprise you.

Suggested Preparation
Music? *He* is the Guardian.

Time Out
Sit facing each other. Hold hands, look into each other's eyes, and take at least five minutes to remember silently all the reasons you have to be grateful to be together. Compose a prayer of gratitude for having your partner in your life. If you wish, speak it out loud.

Activity
- Do this *Activity* seated. Partner A should start by massaging Partner B's hands using a bit of massage oil. First energize your own hands by rubbing them together. Then take your lover's hand and slowly work your way up each finger. Gently pull on each finger. Gently flex and then rotate the wrist. Firmly massage each bit of the surface of the palm. Use your thumb to massage the back of the hand in small circles, too. Now, give special attention to the wrist areas as you massage. End by kissing the hand you have finished.
- While your partner is massaging your hands, describe your first experience of intercourse in as much detail as you wish. Is it a happy memory? What was right about it? What would have made it better? What would have made you feel safer? More loved? More loving? Then, while you do your partner's hands, listen as he/she goes through the same exercise. (If you have never made love, describe your ideal first encounter.)

When you are ready to go to sleep
- Kiss and snuggle as long as the energy is flowing.
- When you decide you are both adequately relaxed, or if it is evening and you are ready to fall asleep, move into "Prayer for Union" (see below). Unite genitals as you lie in scissors (see previous *Exchange*) or bridge position. Do not try to kiss while in "Prayer." Visualize the sexual energy flowing between you from your genitals through your hearts. For at least fifteen minutes, try not to change positions or

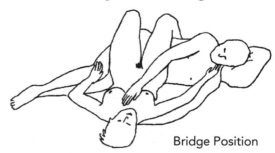

Bridge Position

move, except to get more comfortable (you may find that you have to switch sides or, in rare cases, choose another position on your sides). Express your love with your hands by touching your partner over her heart or placing your hand over his. Relax totally.

↪ Connect as many times as you wish in these positions. If you are overly aroused, gently disconnect, sit up, and circulate energy together. Once you fall asleep, or arise, do not have intercourse again until the *Exchanges* call for it.

Exchange Seventeen:
How Did It Go?

	HIM		HER	
	Yes	No	Yes	No
1. Did you avoid vigorous thrusting?				
2. Did you feel nothing during intercourse and just fall asleep instantly?				
3. Did you find the experience surprisingly satisfying even without thrusting?				
4. Did you kiss and try to heat each other up while in "Prayer"?				
5. Would you be willing to avoid vigorous thrusting if it would protect the loving safety of your relationship?				
6. Did he remain on top of her during the *Exchange*, shortly after it, or at any time since (while naked)?				
7. During or after the *Exchange* did you have the urge to say, "I love you" with words or touch?				
8. Have erotic images of conventional sex or foreplay popped into your mind during, or since, the *Exchange*?				
9. Did you feel totally safe and do you feel comfortable about continuing?				
10. Did you have an orgasm in your sleep afterward?				

The *Key* is on the next page. Check it now.

Key

If you both answered "yes" to the odd-numbered questions and "no" to the even-numbered questions, all is well. If either of you answered two or more of the odd-numbered questions "no" or two or more of the even-numbered questions "yes," then you are trying to go too quickly. Spend more time in the previous Phase. When you feel stable take the *Exchange 15* quiz again with full integrity. When you are ready to proceed, pick up again with *Exchange 15* (substitute *Adventures* from Appendix II for *Activities* already done).

Of course, if you had an orgasm, plan to spend at least two weeks in the Nurturing Phase before picking up with *Exchange 15*.

> NOTE: If at any time as you go forward through the rest of the *Exchanges* erotic images haunt you, consider them a warning. Drop back to the Nurturing Phase for a while.

Let your lovemaking inhale and exhale. Whenever either of you reaches a natural resting place, whether or not you are having intercourse, stop. Most errors at this Phase are made when such natural breathing spaces are ignored.

There is enormous temptation to rush the healing process with forced performance. This is counterproductive, as it triggers uneasiness. Often the temptation is fueled by a desire to please your partner. So make it clear that your pleasure comes from time with your partner rather than his/her performance.

> *Before beginning the* Activity, *talk about what you experienced following the previous* Exchange.

- Do you both feel peaceful today?
- Do you look forward to your activities together? (If not, you are going too fast and need to back up to the previous Phase.)
- What energy movements or joyful sensations did you feel while lying still in "Prayer?" If you insist on moving or kissing during "Prayer" you are still striving to heat yourself up.
- Are you and your lover generous toward each other both in and out of the bedroom? Do even more for your partner.

> *Hey! Did someone have an orgasm? If so, refer to the "Foul-Weather Warning" in the introduction to this Phase.*

Suggested Preparation
Music? *She* is the Guardian.

Time Out
Stand up and enjoy a still, five-minute hug, breathing in through the heart as your partner breathes out through the heart. If you have a shower or hot tub, try this long, still hug there. If you *do* shower as part of the *Time Out,* bathe your lover, not yourself. Let him/her wash you. If you shampoo, do that for each other, too.

Activity
Whoever most enjoys reading out loud reads these quotations to the other. The first is from *Embracing the Beloved,* by Stephen and Ondrea Levine:

> In the beginning of a sexual relationship, each stays in his own body. Rubbing at his edges.... It is two individuals separately having sex, together. If there evolves a meeting of the minds in the body, and the other levels of relationship are in sync with sympathetic intensity, the boundaries break and we pour into each other's space.... Sometimes in lovemaking we have a sense of ourselves disappearing into the other. A sense of ecstatic oneness. Just energy unfolding within the shared spaciousness of being. No *I* or *other.* Nothing separate.[117]

This one is from *Sexual Energy Ecstasy* by David and Ellen Ramsdale*:*

> An aura of peace and benign energy is felt. The best word to describe the feeling is probably sacred. You may feel that you are on truly holy ground. You feel startlingly alive and clearheaded. You feel that the two of you are one.[118]

Has either of you had such a feeling? Share your most inspiring intimate experience with your partner while you hold each other.

When it is time to go to sleep
- ❧ Experiment with different intercourse positions *without intercourse.* Put the emphasis on comfort so you will be able to make love for long periods of time with intervals of stillness. You may wish to try

yab-yum (woman seated in man's lap, facing him) or lying on your sides with the woman's legs wrapped around the man (and supportive pillow arrangements). Or design your own positions.

➤ Choose the most comfortable position you find and be still in it for at least fifteen minutes. Let yourselves relax completely.

➤ If you are feeling a lot of sexual energy moving when you finish, lie still again in scissors or bridge position (see previous *Exchanges* for illustrations). Avoid crawling on top of your partner and passionate kissing. Between now and the next *Exchange,* confine your intimacy to gentle kisses and touches, without intercourse.

NOTE: If you have a tape recorder, prepare for the next *Exchange* by making a meditation tape in advance. The text for the tape appears in the next *Exchange.*

Exchange Eighteen:
Temptation Alert

Temptation is devious. Many of us have the discipline to do the *Exchanges* as written. But once we have finished an *Exchange* there is an urge to go back on autopilot and allow our primitive brains to take the reins. This is especially true if we find ourselves snuggling in between *Exchanges.* Avoid a casual attitude. Your goal is to sidestep sexual hunger and relax into a steady state of wavelike expansion and contraction in your lovemaking. When you have finished this Phase you may discover that you have a workable recipe for the future—one that keeps you attracted to each other but will not lead to fallout. So promise each other now:

➤ If we want to snuggle between *Exchanges* that permit intercourse, we will only go as far as touching genitals in stillness.

➤ Between *Exchanges,* I will not rub around on top of my partner while naked or try to heat my partner up sexually. If I cannot feel a satisfying subtle energy flow between us, I will keep my underwear on so I do not seek to substitute physical gratification for heart energy.

➤ If we miss a day we will begin this Phase again, because experience has shown that these seven *Exchanges,* done on consecutive days, are useful in establishing a new habit.

If at any time you feel that your partner is giving you a double message, speak up. It is all right to note, "You say you are in the mood to make love, but your body says otherwise. How about holding me for a while, and we'll see how we feel later?" Or, "You say you're feeling really satisfied with this approach, but now you're thrusting, or writhing seductively. Have you changed agendas?"

Now, take some time to get clear about your objective. Are you open to further transformation? Are you willing to feel nothing but openhearted compassion for your ex-lovers as well as anyone who ever wronged you? In fact, do you want to see everyone's total innocence despite humankind's madness? These are some of the shifts in perception that accompany this approach to lovemaking. You will grasp what is truly at stake in sexual union. Together you can help end the nasty separation virus infecting humanity.

> *Before beginning the* Activity, *talk about what you experienced following the previous* Exchange.

- ❧ How are you doing with the motionless snuggle in which only energy moves? If you are simply falling asleep the moment you lie still, you are missing the point of this Phase. This time consciously get in touch with your sexual desire, direct it into your lover's heart (without moving), and visualize it coming back to you joined with his or hers. Trust that something is happening even if it is subtle.

- ❧ Have you used the *Exchange 15* signals you worked out for stopping all movement, moving into spoon position, and letting your partner know how much you adore him/her? If not, incorporate them in your snuggling.

> *Pssst! Did someone have an orgasm? If so, refer to the "Foul-Weather Warning" in the introduction to this Phase.*

Suggested Preparation

Find the meditation tape you made or choose some peaceful music. *He* is the Guardian.

Time Out

Sit facing each other (or she can sit in his lap). Place a hand near your lover's heart (or on his back if you are in his lap). With each in-breath, visualize a joyful energy flowing up your spine, through your hand into your lover's heart, and then down to your lover's genitals and back to yours. Do this for several minutes and then relax into stillness for a couple of minutes.

Activity

If you have not prepared a tape in advance, take turns reading the following to each other slowly. Use your imaginations to visualize the images as vividly as possible. The listener/s should sit comfortably with back straight. If possible, hold hands or touch.

Text: *[To be read calmly and slowly with caring. Pause briefly at each ellipsis, and the reader should take a deep, slow breath at each "*".]*

Close your eyes and take long, slow breaths.... Breathe as slowly as possible. *Now, imagine a point at the top of your head.... As you breathe out, allow your awareness to drift from this point down through your body and deep into the earth beneath you.... With each exhalation it drops farther down, like a flat stone settling in fathoms of deep water.

*Now, with each inhalation, imagine you are drawing energy up from deep within the earth.... It is a vibrant, wholesome, nourishing energy.... It glows with the radiant green color of a healthy leaf in sunlight. *Let it flood your body with tingling energy. *You draw it up from the earth, then shower it out from the top of your head and let it fall around you continuously.

*Now, imagine an infinite supply of sparkling, golden light above your head. *Imagine that a gentle ray of this light enters the top of your head with its energizing, healing power. *Begin to glow with this light. *When it has filled your body, let it spread beneath you both, like a puddle, and take the shape of an exquisite golden lotus flower. *It holds you both together in comfort and security.... It heals you.... It balances you.... You both feel full of smiling energy.*

Now, allow the golden light and the green light to swirl together between your two hearts, and expand to envelop you both in a radiant cocoon. *You are one with your partner. . . . Your sense of well-being is so profound that you cannot even remember what it felt like to crave something you missed.*

Now, become aware of your breathing. . . . Allow yourself to retain a sense of your oneness, wholeness, and total vibrant good health. . . . Smile. *And when you are ready, . . . open your eyes and see the Light in each other's eyes.

When it is time to go to sleep:

- ⟿ Snuggle safely for as long as you like.
- ⟿ When you are both adequately relaxed, or if it is evening and you are ready to fall asleep, move into your favorite comfortable position and merely press your genitals together.

Exchange Nineteen:
Self-Love & Selfless Love

 Do you sense changes in yourself since you have been doing the *Exchanges*?

I feel as if I'm awakening from a bad dream. I thought I liked myself, but I certainly didn't like the things I found myself doing. I would watch myself pull away from my partner and think, "There I go again." But I couldn't prevent it. Even though things are already very different I don't feel like I've changed. I feel like I'm just more who I really was. I keep my commitments, I get more done than ever before, and my relationship is going more smoothly than any other. It all feels natural and struggle-free. And now I definitely like who I am.   —Rod

Your partner's loving presence in your life is enough to allow you to function with a greater sense of well-being. You do not need your partner's money or help, though giving always rewards you both. What you really need is the balance and stability attained through mutual caring and closeness. They are the keys to the beneficial changes that accompany this other approach to lovemaking. In other words, you avoid focusing on physical gratification in order to prevent your primitive brain from making you driven and self-centered, or sacrificing and exhausted. A focus on giving and a sense of formality (planned lovemaking) ensure that your relationship continues to thrive.

Many of us have been hooked on the addictiveness of orgasm for so long that we have lost sight of who we really are. As one friend put it, "I now see that it's as if I was taking a drug since I started masturbating at age twelve." By this point in the *Exchanges,* however, your neurochemical responses to intimacy have probably shifted. So the real you is likely to be shining through your former disguise. Acknowledge your sexual magnetism and newfound sense of well-being.

> *Before beginning the* Activity, *talk about what you experienced following the previous* Exchange.

- Since beginning the *Exchanges* have you had intercourse in any position other than scissors, bridge, or *yab-yum* (woman seated in man's lap, facing him)? If so, begin this Phase again. You have derailed.
- Do you both feel ready for intercourse? Have your genitals been aroused enough to connect? If not, begin this Phase again.
- Do you feel a larger purpose in what you are doing together? If so, how would you describe it?

> *Whoops! Did someone have an orgasm? If so, refer to the "Foul-Weather Warning" in the introduction to this Phase.*

Suggested Preparation
Music? *She* is the Guardian.

Time Out
- Have your partner lie on his/her stomach on the bed. Gently, slowly stroke upward from the tailbone to the neck, using hand-over-hand motions. Do it at least three times. Then place one hand on the sacrum and one hand at the top of the spine and rest your hands there for several moments. Can you feel energy flowing between your hands? What does your partner feel?
- Change roles.

Activity
- Discuss what changes you have felt in yourselves, if any, since you began the *Exchanges.*

❧ Each of you reads one of these quotations to the other.

> I will never forget the kiss, never. It opened me up into a rainbow of love, and the pain I felt just vanished. It was like an explosion of emotions fighting to release themselves out of my body into yours. I melted into one with you. It was while we were making love. I could not release nor fight the feeling of freedom. I felt it came close to flying. It never happened before, never... and the orgasm that came later was an anticlimax compared to the feelings I had.
>
> —Anonymous

❧ This one comes from *Sacred Sexuality* by Georg Feuerstein:

> All of a sudden I felt no separation between us.... It was so uncomplicated and natural, and my mind was amazingly calm and quiet.[119]

When it is time to go to sleep

❧ Whoever was the Giving Partner takes the lead. This *Exchange* assumes it is the woman, but if it is the man that is fine.

❧ The Giving Partner uses her kisses, touches, and the gentle movements of her body on top of him or next to him to make him feel loved. Limit direct genital stimulation to the most fleeting and affectionate of gestures, focusing instead on the rest of his body. Make no effort to stimulate an erection. Avoid oral sex. If he grows overly aroused, lie still next to him, synchronize breathing, and gently rest your hand on his penis until he calms down.

❧ See his body as a three-dimensional extension of his spirit. Sense him as a shining light to whom you want to communicate (1) how adored he is, and (2) how honored you feel to be nurturing him and uniting with him. Keep your touch gentle and reverent.

❧ This is an intercourse *Exchange* so, if you are both ready, you may connect genitals and lie still. Choose scissors, bridge, *yab-yum* (woman seated in man's lap, facing him), or woman-on-top position. Have intercourse as often as you like, but keep the movements gentle and avoid deep thrusting. Pause frequently to savor the stillness and more subtle energy flows. Stop when the energy stops flowing for either of you. Make no effort to heat yourselves up.

❧ Should you sense your partner becoming too hot, tensing up, or constricting his breathing, stop, suggest you both circulate your energy, and relax totally. You would do well to ignore your partner's sincere and convincing assurances that he has it all under control. Your intuition is more reliable under such circumstances than his assessment. Likewise, he should keep you away from The Edge and counsel the same countermeasures.

❧ And you, Receiving Partner, remember that your sole responsibility is to relax and enjoy your lover's creative touches and affectionate generosity. Stay seated, or on your back or side, as she directs. And if she directs you to lie on top of her while you are both naked, refuse. She has lost sight of the goal temporarily.

❧ In between *Exchanges* avoid intercourse, though you may always end your snuggling with "Prayer for Union" or some other comfortable position, without intercourse.

Exchange Twenty:
The Bridge

Inspired harmony is an ideal precondition for personal growth, creative solutions, and effortless cooperation with others. By learning to use sex and your relationship to attain inner balance, you gradually quiet the forces within that formerly drove you to seek externally for a sense of satisfaction. And, with fewer power struggles and personality conflicts, you have the time, energy, and resources for assisting others and fulfilling your larger goals.

After a year of making love this other way, one of my friends said, "This has been the happiest period of my life." Happiness heals. It ensures a body chemistry that feels good, stays balanced, and makes you more youthful. When you feel good you also tend to eat better and exercise appropriately. Moreover, happiness increases your confidence, helps you see the humor in things, and lets you focus on solutions rather than problems.

Biology cares nothing for happiness. In its blind drive to replicate your genes, it would have you oscillate between costly indulgence and toxic isolation. Fortunately, you now know there is a middle way that lets you feel totally alive and enjoy making love frequently without setting off a sense of deprivation. Once you experience for yourself this unfamiliar but revitalizing path, you can more easily cope with those who are still brainwashed by biology. You can simply point to the solution to humanity's perennial sense of deprivation with compassion. You become a living example of the benefits of relationships that heal.

According to various esoteric traditions around the world, this simple change in habits is not merely a path to harmony, but also a path to full spiritual awakening—a sort of bridge between human limitation and true liberation. It may be that some of us chose to come back with a lot of sexual energy just so we would discover that the world's proposed solutions for the fallout from biological sex do not work. That realization may at first have been unwelcome, but ultimately it has motivated us to try a better way. So see a larger purpose in your sexual encounters. You may be among the vanguard of a major healing force on the planet.

Inner balance aligns you with a larger flow of energy. That is, you sense more easily where you should be, what you should be doing for the greater good, and with whom. In this regard, you may both have to be willing to share what you have learned with new partners. As unsettling as this concept can be, nothing convinces you of the power of healing sexual relationships more effectively than sharing your ability to heal with another. At last you recognize that your remarkable harmony is, indeed, a product of your new habits, and not of the unique chemistry between you and your current partner. So if you are pulled apart by the giant hand of fate, seize the opportunity to share your gift with another.

Before beginning the Activity, *talk about what you experienced following the previous* Exchange.

- What did you like best that the Giving Partner did? Did anything surprise you? Did you feel adored? Do you feel complete today?
- Did you allow yourselves any periods of stillness to see if you could feel subtle or joyful energy moving? Did you stop making love when the energy stopped flowing, or try to stimulate each other back to another high? Try stopping when the energy stops.
- Do both your bodies easily become aroused? If not, you are going

too quickly. Return to the Nurturing Phase and wait until your bodies are enthusiastic about proceeding, without resorting to conventional foreplay. Was there any vigorous thrusting? If so, begin this Phase again.

ꙮ Which *Activities* or *Time Outs* have each of you liked most? Want to add them to your lovemaking repertoire?

> *Hmmm ... if someone had an orgasm, refer to the "Foul-Weather Warning" in the introduction to this Phase.*

Suggested Preparation
Find blankets or a mat. Music? *He* is the Guardian.

Time Out
Sit facing each other, put a pillow in your laps, and hold each other's elbows or forearms. Touch foreheads and be still for several minutes, breathing through your hearts. Can you feel a subtle ecstasy in your body?

Activity
ꙮ Partner A lies on the floor on a blanket in the position he/she usually curls into when feeling abandoned, unloved, or betrayed. Partner B kneels by his or her head and gently holds it for a moment, eyes closed.

ꙮ Then, with lots of kisses, Partner B slowly takes at least five minutes to untangle Partner A gently, limb by limb, until he/she is resting comfortably on his or her back, palms up, arms and legs straight, but relaxed. Partner B should make a conscious effort to send Partner A healing energy to dissolve all old programming relating to defensive isolation.

ꙮ When Partner B has finished, Partner A thanks Partner B by holding him/her for a while.

ꙮ Switch roles.[120]

When it is time to go to sleep
ꙮ He should use his kisses, touches and desire-to-merge to make her feel loved rather than hot. Relax frequently. Do not connect genitals.

Just allow yourselves to calm down in between periods of arousal.

- ❧ Should you sense your partner becoming too hot, tensing up, or constricting her breathing, stop, suggest you both circulate your energy, and relax totally. She should counsel the same countermeasures if necessary. Stay focused on the flow of energy between you.
- ❧ Even though you are not having intercourse, make love in gentle waves for as long as the energy is flowing for both of you. Stop when it stops for either of you. You may find it calming to lie still in a comfortable intercourse position, but without intercourse.

Exchange Twenty-One:
The Finish Line

This *Exchange* is the last one. So check your *Harmony Index*. It may help you assess whether the *Exchanges* have benefited you. Check off the statements that are true for you, though you may be firmly convinced that the changes have nothing to do with the *Exchanges*. (To be sure, you can only evaluate their effects if you did the *Exchanges* as written.)

Harmony Index
Since we began the *Exchanges*,

HIM	HER	
❏	❏	I'm sleeping better.
❏	❏	I've cut back on, or dropped, an unhealthy addiction.
❏	❏	My health has noticeably improved in some way.
❏	❏	I'm thinking more clearly.
❏	❏	I'm in less pain.
❏	❏	I'm smiling more.
❏	❏	I'm more productive and deal with tough problems more effectively.
❏	❏	The kids are behaving better.
❏	❏	I'm bickering with my partner, in-laws, or bothersome bureaucrats less.
❏	❏	I feel more loved.
❏	❏	I'm watching television less.

❑   ❑   I feel like we'll always be friends whatever happens.
❑   ❑   Aspects of our relationship have healed.
❑   ❑   I'm less broke, exhausted, and rushed.
❑   ❑   My fear of intimacy has decreased.
❑   ❑   I have fewer hassles at work.
❑   ❑   I've lightened up—depressions are less frequent.
❑   ❑   I feel more youthful.
❑   ❑   I seem to be developing more psychic ability.
❑   ❑   I have a sense of optimism about the future.

Do you plan to stick with your new lovemaking habits? It can take months of consistent practice with this new approach to register the full advantages. If you decide to return to your old habits, you may want to check this index again in a month to see how many of the statements above are true for you then.

Remember, we were never kicked out of paradise. We have just thoroughly ignored its presence thanks to our vibration-lowering, grabbing, sacrificing, and isolating mentalities of the past. The costs of conventional sex have been far greater than we realize, and the rewards of changing our ways are, too.

For the Future

Tomorrow is an intercourse day. So practice all your new skills with total integrity and an extra dose of caution. It is very easy to fall back into old habits once you leave your drills behind.

✤ If you decide to stick with your new lovemaking habits, *stay on your schedule*. Remember:

- Make love only once per day, and not every day.
- If you do not have intercourse on a scheduled occasion, avoid it the next day as well. Give your nervous system a chance to calm down completely. Constant desire will erode your equilibrium.
- If you have been apart for days, delay intercourse at least until your second day together.
- If you decide to be spontaneous now and then, wait your scheduled interval before your next occasion.

- While spoon position is great for comforting your partner or falling asleep together, it is not recommended for intercourse. It can be emotionally alienating and leave too much focus on physical gratification.
- Even when you are tired or busy, try to include a five-minute generous exchange before you go to sleep, either in the form of a *Time Out* or in the form of a brief head, face, foot, chest, back, ear, or other massage. It can give you energy.
- When you move during intercourse, move gently and consciously. Avoid deep thrusts, as they tend to escalate your lovemaking and allow impulse to take over.
- Include periods of stillness in your snuggling and lovemaking. An experience of true merging can only happen when your consciousness expands beyond physical sensation.
- It is a good idea to do the *Exchanges* periodically to reorient your lovemaking. Which month would you make "Exchanges Month"?

Before beginning the Activity, *talk about what you experienced following the previous* Exchange.

- How did it feel to have your lover gently untangle you from your "miserable" position? Do you think the feeling of being comforted will stay with you?
- By contrast, do you think you have reached an impasse? If so, you may find the checklist in Appendix I useful.

Yoohoo! Did someone have an orgasm? If so, refer to the "Foul-Weather Warning" in the introduction to this Phase.

Suggested Preparation
Music? *She* is the Guardian.

Time Out
- Sit next to your partner, who is lying next to you. Place one hand over the heart and one hand over the belly. As your partner breathes in, you breathe out through your heart, sending him/her the energy of radiant good health.
- Change roles.

Activity

- ❧ Whoever most enjoys reading aloud reads these quotations to the other. The first one comes from *Taoist Secrets of Love: Cultivating Male Sexual Energy.*

It is a state of prolonged orgasm. . . . It is a fusion of opposites, a meltdown. . . . This releases a tremendous energy that is truly thrilling as it radiates out to fill every cell of your body and joins it together with your lover.[121]

I was very open, relaxed and clear, and she who was with me seemed to be in a similar state: a joint experiencing of inner quietude, a great deal of attention for one another and a great intensity. And as the excitement increased, the state of relaxation only deepened, and, like a river, the emotion ran into an ocean of peace, expanding it continuously. The more excited I was the more transparent consciousness became. The flow of energy causing an ever-deepening inner peace! Rather than "climbing the mountain," I more and more became a valley. Expansion had replaced the common contraction mechanism. —H. Stiekema

- ❧ Take turns asking each other, "What do I do that makes you feel most loved?" If it is convenient do it now.

When it is time to go to sleep

- ❧ Snuggle gently and reverently. Hold your partner tightly and silently thank him/her for sharing the *Exchanges* with you.
- ❧ Pray for or visualize a strong, healthy, balanced relationship for the two of you, one that can serve as a reliable vessel for a joy-filled voyage of personal and spiritual growth.

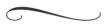

Thanks for trying the *Exchanges.*
Send an email to feedback@reuniting.info to share your experiences in healing relationships with others.

Notes

1. Barbara Dafoe Whitehead and Dave Popenoe, "The State of Our Unions: The Social Health of Marriage in America 2001," The National Marriage Project, Rutgers, the State University of New Jersey (June 2001): 10, 15.
2. Ibid.
3. D.F. Fiorino, et al., "Dynamic Changes in Nucleus Accumbens Dopamine Efflux During the Coolidge Effect in Male Rats," *Journal of Neuroscience* 17:12 (June 15, 1997): 4849–4855.
4. Terry Burnham and Jay Phelan, *Mean Genes: From Sex to Money to Food, Taming Our Primal Instincts* (New York: Penguin Putnam Inc., 2000): 184–185.
5. F. B. Furlow and R. Thornhill, "The orgasm wars (adaptive function of the female orgasm)," *Psychology Today* 29(1996): 42–46.
6. R. Thornhill, et al., "Human female orgasm and mate fluctuating asymmetry." *Animal Behavior* 50 (1995): 1601–1615. R. Thornhill and A.P. Moller. "Developmental stability, disease, and medicine." *Biological Reviews of the Cambridge Philosophical Society* 72 (1997): 497–548.
7. Richard Dawkins, *The Selfish Gene* (Oxford: Oxford University Press, 1976): 22.
8. Leo Tolstoy, *The Kreutzer Sonata* (Chapter 2) See http://etext.lib.virginia.edu/toc/modeng/public/TolKreu.html. Note: Helen's attraction to Paris caused the Trojan War.
9. Mantak Chia and Manewan Chia, *Healing Love Through the Tao* (Huntington: Healing Tao Books, 1986): 291.
10. Ed. Diana Trilling, *The Portable D. H. Lawrence* (New York: Penguin Books, 1977): 654.
11. John Lee, *The Flying Boy* (Deerfield Beach, FL: Health Communications, Inc., 1989): 10.
12. Trans. and ed. James Freud and Anna Freud, *The Future of an Illusion; Civilization and Its Discontents; and Other Works, The Standard Edition of the Complete Psychological Works of Sigmund Freud,* vol. 21 (London: The Hogarth Press and the Institute of Psychological Analysis, 1968): 154.
13. Mantak Chia, *Taoist Secrets of Love: Cultivating Male Sexual Energy* (Santa Fe: Aurora Press, 1984): 44.
14. Herb Goldberg, PhD. *What Men Really Want* (New York: New American Library, 1991): 112.
15. Keith Dowman, *Sky Dancer: The Secret Life and Songs of the Lady Yeshe Tsogyel* (London: Routledge and Kegan Paul, 1984): 248.
16. Sally Cline, *Women, Passion & Celibacy* (New York: Carol Southern Books, 1993): 91. See also *Sensual Celibacy* by Donna Marie Williams, and *Solitaire: The Intimate Lives of Single Women* by Marian Botsford Fraser.
17. Herb Goldberg Ph.D., *What Men Really Want* (New York: New American Library, 1991): 77.

18. Barry Long, "Making Love: Sexual Love the Divine Way" audio tape (Barry Long Books, 1996).

19. Swami Satyananda Saraswati, *Kundalini Tantra* (Bihar: Bihar School of Yoga, 1992).

20. Nicole Christine, *Temple of the Living Earth* (Sedona: Earth Song Publications, 1995): 18,19.

21. Quoted in "Life without Sex" (*Yoga Journal,* November 2002): 99.

22. Edgar Cayce Reading No: 3686–1, M.65, quoted in *Sex and the Spiritual Path* by Herbert B. Puryear (Virginia Beach: A.R.E. Press, 1980): 144.

23. R. Baker and M.A. Bellis, *Human Sperm Competition: Copulation, Masturbation, and Infidelity* (New York: Chapman & Hall, 1995): 197.

24. "Scent of a Man," *New Scientist* (February 10, 2001), www.skyaid.org%20Org/Medical/scent_of_a_man.htm.

25. Robin Baker, *Sperm Wars: Infidelity, Sexual Conflict and Other Bedroom Battles* (Basingstokes Hampshire: MacMillan Publishers Ltd., 2002).

26. Terry Burnham and Jay Phelan, *Mean Genes: From Sex to Money to Food, Taming Our Primal Instincts* (New York: Penguin USA, 2001)

27. Ibid., p. 64.

28. H. Fisher, et al., "Lust, Attraction, Attachment: Defining the brain systems for love with an emphasis on the neural circuitry of romantic attraction," *Journal of Sex and Marital Therapy* 31(5) (October 2002).

29. D.E. Riley, "Reversible transvestic fetishism in a man with Parkinson's Disease," *Clinical Neuropharmacology* 25(4) (Jul-Aug. 2002): 234–237.

30. Steven R. Quartz and Terrence J. Sejnowski, *Liars, Lovers and Heroes* (New York: HarperCollins Publishers, Inc., 2002): 109.

31. Ibid.

32. Janice Kiecolt-Glaser, et al., "Marital Stress: Immunological, Endocrinological and Health Consequences," *Psychology and Medicine,* Ohio State University College of Medicine, http://pni.psychiatry.ohio-state.edu/jkg/newlywed.htm.

33. Gilles Marin, *Healing from Within with Chi Nei Tsang* (Berkeley: North Atlantic Books, 1999): 143.

34. S.P. Yang, et al., "Involvement of endogenous opioidergic neurons in modulation of prolactin secretion in response to mating in the female rat" (*MEDLINE,* 2000).

35. P. Haake, et al., "Absence of orgasm-induced prolactin secretion in a healthy multi-orgasmic male subject," *International Journal of Impotence Research* 14(2) (April 2002): 133–135.

36. G.A. Maquire, "Prolactin elevation with antipsychotic medications: mechanisms of action and clinical consequences," *Journal of Clinical Psychiatry* 63, Suppl. 4 (2002): 56–62.

37. Mantak Chia, *Taoist Secrets of Love: Cultivating Male Sexual Energy* (Sante Fe: Aurora Press, 1984): 46.

38. Daniel Goleman, *Emotional Intelligence* (New York: Bantam Books, 1995): 17.

39. Helen Fisher, "Lust, Attraction, and Attachment in Mammalian Reproduction," *Human Nature* 9(1) (1998).

40. Kate Egan, "Love & Sex: The Vole Story," *Emory Medicine* (Summer 1998), quoting T.R Insel, neruoscientist and director of the Yerkes Regional Primate Center.

41. M.L. Boccia and C.A. Pedersen, "Oxytocin maintains as well as initiates female sexual behavior: effects of a highly selective oxytocin antagonist," *Horm. Behav.* 41(2) (March 2002): 170–177.

42. A.C. Harmon, et al., "Social experience and social context alter the behavioral response to centrally administered oxytocin in female Syrian hamsters," *Neuroscience* 109(4) (2002): 767–772.

43. G. Gimpl and F. Fahrenholz, "The oxytocin receptor system: structure, function, and regulation," *Physiol Rev.* 81(2) (April 2001): 629–683.

44. G. Ironson, et al., "Massage Therapy is Associated with Enhancement of the Immune System's Cytotoxic Capacity," *International Journal of Neuroscience* 84(1–4) (1996): 205–217.

45. Therapeutic effects of massage taken from Mosby's *Fundamentals of Therapeutic Massage, 2d ed.,* Sandy Fritz (Harcourt Health Sciences Company, 2000): 150–154.

46. E.B. Palrnore, "Predictors of the Longevity Difference: A 25-year Follow-up," *Gerontologist* 6 (1982): 513–518.

47. L.A. Abramov, "Sexual Life and Frigidity among Women Developing Acute Myocardial Infarction," *Psychosomatic Medicine* 38 (1976): 418–425.

48. Davey Smith, et al., "Sex and Death: Are they related? Findings from the Caerphilly Cohort Study," *British Medical Journal* 315, No: 7123 (1997):1641–1644.

49. Jack Chellem, "The Prediabetic Epidemic: Syndrome X is a relatively new diagnosis, but it is a condition as old as the typical American diet," *Nutrition Science News* (March 2001).

50. S.S. Knox, et al., "Social isolation and cardiovascular disease: an atherosclerotic pathway?" *Psychoneuroendocrinology* 23(8) (1998): 877–890.

51. J.H.K.C. Medalie, et al., "Angina Pectoris among 10,000 Men," *American Journal of Medicine* 60(6) (1976): 910–921.

52. Dean Ornish, M.D., *Love & Survival* (New York: HarperCollins Publishers, 1998): 2, 3.

53. Press release entitled "Hormone Involved in Reproduction May Have A Role in the Maintenance of Relationships," University of California, San Francisco (July 15, 1999).

54. See both S.S. Cui, et al., "Prevention of cannabinoid withdrawal syndrome by lithium: involvement of oxytocinergic neuronal activation," *Journal of Neuroscience* 21(24) (December 2001): 9867–9876., and Kovacs, et al., "Oxytocin and Addiction: A Review," *Psychoneuroendocrinology* 23(8) (November 1998): 945–962.

55. Robert Coombs, "Marital Status and Personal Well-Being: A Literature Review," *Family Relations* 40 (1991): 97–102.

56. R.K. Ross, et al., "A Cohort Study of Mortality from Cancer of the Prostate in Catholic Priests," *British Journal of Cancer* 43(2) (1981): 233–235.

57. Linda Waite, "Does Marriage Matter?" *Demography* 32(1995): 483–507.

58. Horwitz, et al., "Becoming Married and Mental Health: A Longitudinal Study of a Cohort of Young Adults," *Journal of Marriage and the Family* 58 (1997): 895–907.

59. Catherine E. Ross, "Reconceptualizing Marital Status as a Continuum of Social Attachment," *Journal of Marriage and the Family* 57 (1995): 129–140.

60. Lillard and Waite, "'Til Death Do Us Part': Marital Disruption and Mortality," *American Journal of Sociology* 100(5) (1995): 1131–1156.

61. Daniel Goleman, *Emotional Intelligence* (New York: Bantam Books, 1995): 178, citing James House, et al., "Social Relationships and Health," *Science* (July 29, 1988).

62. J. Allman, et al., "Parenting and survival in anthropoid primates: Caretakers live longer," *Proceedings of the National Academy of Sciences USA* 95 (1998): 6866–6869.

63. Nancy Deutsch, "'Tis Healthier to Give than to Receive," *HealthScoutNews* (November 26, 2002).

64. Allan Luks, "Helper's high: volunteering makes people feel good, physically and emotionally," *Psychology Today* (Oct. 1988): 40.

65. Rollin McCraty, et al., "Science of the Heart: Research Overview and Summaries," HeartMath Research Center, Institute of HeartMath (No. 01–001, 2001), Web site: http://www.heartmath.org.

66. Doc Childre and Howard Martin, *The HeartMath Solution* (San Francisco: HarperSanFrancisco, 1999): 160.

67. Daniel Goleman, *Emotional Intelligence* (New York: Bantam Books, 1995): 81.

68. Sandra R. Leiblum, PhD, "Sexual Problems and Dysfunction: Epidemiology, Classification, and Risk Factors," *Journal of Gender-Specific Medicine* 2(5) (1999): 41–45.

69. John Gray, Ph.D., *Mars and Venus in the Bedroom* (New York: HarperCollins, 1997): 19.

70. Adi Da Samraj, ed. Meg McDonnell, *The Scale of the Very Small,* quoting from *Love of the Two-Armed Form* (The Ruchira Buddha Foundation Pty Ltd, 1997): 118.

71. Marilyn Elias, "Stress eases after age 60, even for overtaxed women," *USA Today* (Saturday, August 24, 2002) reporting on study by David Almeida, Ph.D. of the University of Arizona.

72. William Bloom, *The Endorphin Effect* (London: Piatkus Books, 2001).

73. Willard F. Harley, Jr., *Love Busters* (Grand Rapids: Baker Book House Company, 2002): 35, 37.

74. http://www.oprah.com/tows/pastshows/tows_2000/tows_past/ 20000222.jhtml. Also see, *OK, So I Don't Have a Headache* by Christina Ferrare and *I'm Not in the Mood* by Judith Reichman.

75. "Number, Timing and Duration of Marriages and Divorces: 1996," issued February 2002, Census Bureau, *Current Population Reports:* 18.

76. Janice Kiecolt-Glaser, et al., "Marital Stress: Immunological, Endocrinological and Health Consequences," *Psychology and Medicine,* Ohio State University College of Medicine, http://pni.psychiatry.ohio-state.edu/jkg/newlywed.htm.

77. Orth-Gome'r, et al., "The Stockholm Female Coronary Risk Study," *Journals of the AMA* 284(23) (2000).

78. James Coyne, M.D., et al., "Prognostic importance of marital quality for survival of congestive heart failure," *American Journal of Cardiology* 88 (2001): 526–529.

79. Tucker, et al., "Marital History at Midlife as a Predictor of Longevity: Alternative Explanations to the Protective Effect of Marriage," *Health Psychology* 15:2 (1996): 94–101.

80. H. Morowitz, "Hiding in the Hammond Report," *Hospital Practice* (1975): 39.

81. Barry Duncan Psy.D. and Joseph Rock Psy.D., *Face It, Men Are @$$H%c$! What Women Can Do About It* (Deerfield Beach, FL: Health Communications, 1998).

82. "Marital Status and Living Arrangements: March 1996," issued March 1998, Census Bureau, *Current Population Reports:* 1.

83. "Number, Timing and Duration of Marriages and Divorces: 1996," issued February 2002, Census Bureau, *Current Population Reports:* 18.

84. Barbara Dafoe Whitehead and Dave Popenoe, "The State of Our Unions: The Social Health of Marriage in America 2001, Who Wants To Marry A Soul Mate?: New Survey Findings on Young Adults' Attitudes about Love and Marriage," The National Marriage Project, Rutgers, the State University of New Jersey: 8, 5.

85. Harold W. Percival, *Thinking and Destiny* (Dallas: The Word Publishing Company, 1946): 169–171.

86. D.E. Riley, "Reversible transvestic fetishism in a man with Parkinson's disease treated with selegiline," *Clinical Neuropharmacol.* 25(4) July–August 2002): 234–237.

87. Edgar Cayce, Reading 262–86, A.R.E., Virginia Beach, VA.

88. Harold W. Percival, *Thinking and Destiny* (Dallas: The Word Foundation, Inc., 1946): 59.

89. Edgar Cayce, Reading 3704–1, F.23, quoted in *Sex and the Spiritual Path* by Herbert B. Puryear (Virginia Beach: A.R.E. Press, 1980): 183.

90. Being Peace, from the compilation *The Wisdom of Thich Nhat Hanh* (New York: One Spirit, by arrangement with Beacon Press and Parallex Press, 2000): 251.

91. Stag-sam Nus-ldan-rdo-rje, trans. and com. Keith Dowman, *Sky Dancer: The Secret Life and Songs of the Lady Yeshe Tsogyel* (London: Routledge and Kegan Paul, 1984): 230, 249.

92. Padm Sambhava, trans. and com. Keith Dowman, *The Legend of the Great Stupa and The Life Story of the Lotus-Born Guru* (Berkeley: Dharma Publishing, 1973).

93. Barbara Dafoe Whitehead and Dave Popenoe, "The State of Our Unions: The Social Health of Marriage in America 2001, Who Wants To Marry A Soul Mate?: New Survey Findings on Young Adults' Attitudes about Love and Marriage," The National Marriage Project, Rutgers, the State University of New Jersey: 1, 5.

94. The Electronic Version of *A Course in Miracles,* (CenterLink Information Services, Inc. under an agreement with the copyright holder, the Foundation for Inner Peace, 1975) T–20.IV.6.

95. Ibid. T–22.VI.4.

96. Ibid. T–17.IV.1, T–5.in.1.

97. Ibid. T–3.VII.4.

98. Ibid. T–18.II.6, T–21.III.12.

99. Ibid. W–155.4–5.

100. Ibid. T–22.IV.1.

101. Ibid. T–22.VI.1.

102. Ibid. T–26.II.7.

103. Ibid. T–29.I.6.
104. Ibid. T–27.VII.2, T–27.VIII.8.
105. Ed. Andrew Welburn, *Gnosis, the Mysteries and Christianity* (Edinburgh: Floris Books, 1994): 287.
106. Ibid.
107. Jorunn Jacobsen Buckley, "The Holy Spirit is a Double Name: Holy Spirit, Mary, Sophia in the Gospel of Philip," from *Images of the Feminine in Gnosticism,* ed. Karen L. King (Fortress Press Philadelphia for Studies in Antiquity and Christianity, 1988): 227.
108. Trans. Wesley W. Isenberg, *The Gospel of Phillip,* Wesley Center Online, Applied Theology, Northwest Nazarene University (1993–2002), http://weley.nnu.edu/noncanon/gospels/gosphil.htm.
109. Ibid.
110. Trans. Wesley W. Isenberg, *The Gospel of Thomas,* Ed. James M. Robinson, *The Nag Hammadi Library* (San Francisco: Harper Collins Publishers, 3rd Edition, 1988): 129.
111. Mary Sharpe, "Sexuality and the Sacred in Gnostic Literature," Dissertation (University of Cambridge, Faculty of Theology and Religious Studies) 2001.
112. Adi Da Samraj, ed. Meg McDonnell, *The Scale of the Very Small,* quoting from *Love of the Two-Armed Form* (The Ruchira Buddha Foundation Pty Ltd, 1997): 117–118.
113. Alice A. Bailey and the Tibetan Master, Djwhal Khul, *A Compilation On Sex* (New York: Lucis Publishing Company, 1980): 75, 81.
114. Lao Tzu, *Hua Hu Ching,* trans. Brian Walker (New York: HarperCollins Publishers, 1992): §69, p. 88.
115. Michael D. Birnbaum, M.D., "Pregnancy and Frequency of Intercourse." http://www.infertilityphysician.com/ovulation/pregnancy.html.
116. This potent suggestion comes from Doc Childre and Howard Martin, authors of *The HeartMath Solution* (San Francisco: HarperCollins, 1999).
117. Stephen and Ondrea Levine, *Embracing the Beloved: Relationship As a Path of Awakening* (New York: Anchor Books, 1996): 161–162.
118. David and Ellen Ramsdale, *Sexual Energy Ecstasy* (New York: Bantam Doubleday Dell, 1993): 362.
119. Georg Feuerstein, *Sacred Sexuality* (New York: Jeremy P. Tarcher/Perigee, 1993).
120. I was first introduced to a form of this exercise at Findhorn, a spiritual community in Scotland.
121. Mantak Chia, *Taoist Secrets of Love: Cultivating Male Sexual Energy* (Sante Fe: Aurora Press, 1984): 154.

Appendix I:
Impasse Checklist

If you have a sense that something is not right, fear may still be undermining your efforts. After all, you began the *Exchanges* with your Intimacy Sabotaging Device fully operational. While the *Exchanges* are an effective way to deactivate it, you may be resisting their gifts without even realizing it.

What if you honestly suspect you have achieved all you can together? Here is a checklist to help you decide if you have reached an impasse.

HIM   HER

❏   ❏   One of you had an orgasm. Even so, you continued with the *Exchanges* instead of backing up and waiting two weeks *and* until you could honestly answer the *Exchange 15* questions necessary to move safely into intercourse. [If you checked this box you need look no further for the cause of your disharmony. Just drop into the Nurturing Phase again and follow directions. Do not assess your compatibility until you have completed the *Exchanges*.]

❏   ❏   There is a growing feeling of uneasy tension between you that does not abate.

❏   ❏   Anger is erupting regularly.

❏   ❏   One of you constantly finds excuses not to do the *Exchanges,* or is totally resistant to the idea of doing them.

❏   ❏   One of you is demanding separation.

❏   ❏   One of you has returned to an old addiction, disappears for entire nights to pursue it, and is making no effort to stop.

❏   ❏   You realize that you are engaging in separation-producing behavior and cannot help yourself.

❏   ❏   You are pushing your partner past the proposed physical intimacy limits of the *Exchanges.*

❏   ❏   The thought of increased intimacy does not appeal to you. In four weeks you have not yet felt the desire for intercourse itself, while your partner clearly does.

❏   ❏   You believe that your partner is not being honest with him-self/herself in some way. Perhaps he/she is just going through the motions without participating fully.

If either of you checked off any of these items (without checking the first one), it could be time to call it quits as lovers for now, and chalk up another relationship crash to the effectiveness of your Intimacy Sabotaging Device. Even if this relationship ends, do not give up. Your loving nourishment of the opposite sex is needed. Try again in the future.

The items listed above point to some of the common ways we sab-otage our efforts to get closer. They are merely symptoms of leftover fear. They do not indicate hopeless character flaws.

Perhaps you have not dismantled your core belief that a partner will never meet your needs or will inevitably abandon you. If so, you may be pushing your partner past healthy limits, or whining about feeling unloved to trigger a rejection. Or you could be bullying your partner into reverting to past habits. Or perhaps you are pulling away on some level instead of nourishing your partner to the best of your ability. Maybe you are holding back because you have not forgiven the oppo-site sex completely for past unhappiness. Or maybe you imagine that you would rather be with someone else. Or perhaps you have an addic-tion to a substance, or to hot sex, that you would rather not let go of just yet.

You would be wise to face these barriers and release the uneasiness underlying these maneuvers with your current partner, if possible. You certainly will not avoid having to clear your discomfort by changing partners. It will show up again.

Whatever your results on the *Impasse Checklist,* take at least three days to think about your decision before abandoning the *Exchanges.* Do *Exchanges 1* or *2* each night while you reflect. Resist the urges to demand your space or go into sensual overdrive. During your nightly contact silently ask for:

•◉ signs to help you decide for the best, and

•◉ insights to help you release your ingrained defenses against intimacy.

Also reflect on the good that has come out of your time together. Have you healed in some respect? Have you successfully passed through any crises and found that your loving feelings returned a couple of weeks afterward? You can do this again. An opportunity to heal each other is precious and should not be discarded lightly just because of an uncomfortable period. Sometimes breakthroughs will surprise you just when you are sure you have stalled out.

If, after three days, either of you feels you can go no further, be content with what you have achieved together. Lovingly release each other with good will. Accept that you may have to work out your debilitating fear with another partner. It is better to face the possibility that the two of you are not destined to be lovers just now and revert to a loving friendship than to force yourself closer, or redesign the *Exchanges* to fit your imagined needs for more emotional distance or more physical gratification.

Appendix II:
Adventures

Nurturing
Get your partner's favorite snack and feed him/her.

Poetry
Take turns reading each other your favorite love poem out loud. Then take turns reading your partner's favorite to him/her.

Horseplay
How long has it been since you had an uncontrollable fit of the giggles? Since you allowed yourself to be tickled silly? Since you leg-wrestled, arm-wrestled, or even thumb-wrestled your partner into submission (cheating *allowed*)? Since you had a pillow fight? Since you played hide-and-seek with each other in the dark? Since you picked your partner up and swung her around? Since you hid behind a door and said "Boo!" as your partner went through it? Since you held hands and spun each other around until you collapsed together in dizzy laughter? Or knocked your partner over backward onto the bed and "attacked" him/her enthusiastically? Or, if physically incapacitated, read dumb jokes to each other until you gasped with laughter?

Such activities could prove vital to restoring a spontaneous flow of loving feelings. They raise your spirits, peel off your armor, evict you from your unsuspected ruts, and release beneficial hormones into your bloodstream. You are literally heightening your awareness by carrying on this way. The next day, food tastes better, colors are brighter, and music touches you more deeply. Your partner's smile takes on new radiance. His hugs satisfy more. The way she moves delights you more for no apparent reason. And new pranks come to mind. . . . So, play together with the goal of promoting silly laughter, mock outrage, and enthusiastic revenge.

> NOTE: If this *Activity* brings up uneasiness for either partner, the partner who is uneasy should take the lead and the other partner should be very gentle. Notice your feelings and talk about them.

Service

Take turns asking each other, "How may I serve you?" You may respond with requests that can be carried out immediately, or at the server's discretion. If your request is for touch, only request services that would not carry you beyond the level of physical intimacy you have already reached in the *Exchanges*.

Powder Massage

Light some candles, scent the room, and take turns giving each other a gentle massage using bath powder rather than oil.

Meditation

Try a favorite meditation with your foreheads together, either sitting cross-legged or lying on your sides with your feet at opposite ends of the bed or floor.

Star Gazing

Take a walk at night, holding hands, and stop to look at the night sky together.

Practical

Choose a project that one of you has been procrastinating about and get started on it together. Put on your favorite music and take lots of kissing breaks.

Sharing

Take turns talking about the following:
- Your most "wicked" childhood prank
- Your most disastrous, or funniest, sexual experience
- Your most moving non-genital sexual experience
- Your highest expectations for intimacy between male and female

Going Beyond Roles

Sit facing each other and look into each other's eyes. Decide who will go first. The other partner can close his/her eyes and relax completely with a couple of deep breaths. Hold hands. Now, ask your partner, "Who are you?" Let your partner answer, but without defining himself/herself by reference to any physical attributes. Acknowledge the reply with an "OK," and then sincerely ask the question again. Stop when your intuition tells you that your partner has reached as deep a level of self-definition as possible. Switch roles.

Tomorrow, do some things that are not "you." Take a different path to a regular destination. Go work out, meditate, or read a newspaper, or do not if you normally would. Join your partner's routine at a time you normally would not. Turn off the television for a while and sit with one another, enjoying the silence.

Time Out
Rent a movie, make popcorn, and curl up together.

It's a Beautiful Life
Get comfortable and spend time imagining how the world would be if you had not decided to reincarnate this time around. How would your loved ones' lives have been different? When you finish, think about why you might have decided to return this time. What have you really come to achieve? Talk about what occurs to you.

Bathing Together
If you are both at least two weeks beyond your last genital orgasm, have begun the Healing Phase, and have a bathtub, hot tub, or large shower, try bathing or soaking together. If bathing, be sure to wash your lover rather than yourself. If you shampoo, do that for each other, too. If something needs shaving try shaving your partner.

Spiritual Reading
Take turns reading each other your favorite inspirational material. Does either of you feel differently afterward? Talk about the material.

Sharing Victories
Make a fire and warm drinks (or some cozy equivalent). Tell each other about your finest accomplishments.

Harmony
Listen to vocal (even opera) duets by a man and woman or watch couples ice-skating (Olympic-style).

Stretching

Do yoga or other stretching together (you can each do your own thing) for at least a half hour. Take kissing breaks.

Backing Up

Take turns giving each other a massage back-to-back, with no hands.

Pasta Night

Feed each other spaghetti or noodles with no cutlery.

Comfort

Cradle or hold your partner as if she/he were a daughter or son and be still.

Shoulder Rub

Tell your partner something(s) you really like about your time with him/her while you rub his or her shoulders for a couple of minutes. Switch roles.

Serenade

Sing a love song to your partner. Ham it up. Switch roles. Sing a duet.

Boat and Pilot

He stands behind her and places his hands on her shoulders. She closes her eyes and keeps them closed. For several minutes he pilots her around the room at different speeds. Her role is to trust and relax. His is to be a safe and confident pilot.

Foot Massage with a Twist

- Partner A, lie comfortably on your stomach, on a mat on the floor, with hands palm-down near your head. Be prepared to let your lover know what feels good with wordless sounds and sighs.
- B, stand next to A and use your bare *foot* to massage A gently, consciously sending loving energy through your foot. Begin by placing your foot on one of A's hands. Gently rock some of your weight onto it. Repeat, slowly moving up the fleshy part of A's arms to where the shoulders and neck connect, and then across the shoul-

ders. Then travel around A's body, using a chair to balance your-self as needed. Remember to stand on the soles of A's feet for a moment, too.

- Experiment with a gentle rocking motion that allows A to exhale as your weight descends. And hold the pressure gently but firmly when you feel (or hear) your partner requesting more. You can increase the weight you put on A as A relaxes. Focus on fleshy parts, avoiding the head, spine, shins, elbows, and knees.
- Switch roles.

Index

About the Author

Marnia Robinson earned her B.A. in History at Brown University and her law degree from Yale University. She practiced law for ten years, most recently as Director of Legal Services-Europe at Campbell's Soup. Currently she writes and speaks on relationships and lives in Ashland, Oregon with her husband, Gary Wilson. She invites the reader to contribute insights and experiences at her website, www.reuniting.info.

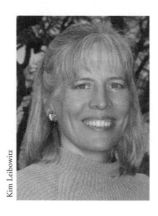

Kim Leibowitz